WALKING,
A MOVING
EXPERIENCE

WALKING,
A MOVING
EXPERIENCE

Herbert W. Hobler

Library of Congress Control Number: 2017913552
ISBN: Hardcover   978-1-5434-4870-2
                 Softcover   978-1-5434-4869-6
                 eBook   978-1-5434-4868-9

Print information available on the last page.

Rev. date: 09/18/2017

To order additional copies of this book, contact:
Xlibris
1-888-795-4274
www.Xlibris.com
Orders@Xlibris.com
766192

CONTENTS

To
Gordon,
Nugget, and Echo
. . . in that order–
And Bonnie for typing
and helping me organize this book.

INTRODUCTION

"Why do I walk? Very simple. I love it. Sure, it's healthy. Sure, it improves your cholesterol count. Sure, it makes your heart beat strong and smooth. More and more doctors prescribe it, but I have never taken a jaunt just because it was healthy. Frankly, I don't like exercise that cuts me off from life."

—Harrison E. Salisbury,
The Good Health Magazine article from
"The New York Times Magazine," April 16, 1989

"No more jogging" were the three words that changed my life 10 years ago. It started one May night in 1981 when I asked my good friend and house guest Gordon Fuqua to jog with me the next morning and he responded "No more jogging since my by-pass, Herb. I walk instead."

The next morning my Golden Retriever Nugget and I joined Gordon on an hour's walk. We heard birds singing. Together we smelled newly mown grass, stopped in the 24-hour WAWA store to buy fresh croissants and a newspaper. We fantasized about the shape of cloud patterns. We saw things in my hometown I had never noticed before. We stopped and chatted for a moment with an acquaintance. We waved at a frenzied jogger who refused to stop and visit. A whole new world of touching, hearing, smelling, meditation and creative thinking opened up before me, one that totally had escaped me as an intense never-stop jogger. Walking was a new adventure—and it was fun!

Within days my pre-breakfast walk became habit. For the next fifteen months I walked four or five days a week. By September 1982 I vowed to thereafter never miss my morning ritual. I bought a pedometer, kept track of my daily walking mileage (most of which was before breakfast), posted my daily mileage on the refrigerator, recorded my weight regularly, and planned a different route every single day. It took more than 800 days of creative planning before I repeated exactly the same route.

By the time I got to my office I felt almost exhilarated. My whole outlook on facing each day was changed by the stimulation of the early morning walk. Subsequently I read an article that medically confirmed what I had already concluded: early morning exercise gets the vital juices going in body and mind.

The idea of never missing at least a one mile walk before breakfast became a fetish. Nothing, I decided, would stand in my way—not weather, nor fatigue, nor aches and pains, nor late hours, not even flying in an airplane. Early mornings are cool, peaceful, and quiet. Dust and smog have yet to appear. Problems later in the day can squelch the best of daily intentions to walk, but an alarm clock can always make time before breakfast.

35,000 miles (including miles before and after breakfast), 15 worn out pairs of shoes, and almost 17 years later, the exhilaration of these morning walks still holds. Over 6,000 consecutive pre-breakfast daily walks have taken me to every part of my Princeton, New Jersey hometown, to 28 states and 26 foreign lands. Normally walking 3½ to 5 miles, my minimum mileage before breakfast has been at least one mile no matter the condition. For 177 consecutive months I never walked less than 150 miles a month, one time reaching 242 miles (while on a walking tour abroad). Never missing a walk before breakfast for 17 years may seem more than a trifle compulsive. Perhaps it is, but that ritual has provided incomparable rewards.

My constant companion and dearest friend for all home town walks for many years was Nugget, my lovable, devoted Golden Retriever. When 13-year-old Nugget passed on, bouncy swift-running Echo became my second Golden Retriever companion. Watching them run free or on leash is always a special joy.

Others may not persevere so consistently nor have the author's privilege of special adventures while traveling broadly for business and pleasure. Still, for every walker, whether of limited or unlimited physical capability, the wonderment of the world is out there—-sunrises, aromas, sounds, the sparkle of the sun on warm water and crusty snow, the adventure of exploring new neighborhoods and distant places.

Everyone agrees that walking improves blood pressure and makes for a trimmer body. But that's only a by-product compared to the stimulation of the mind and the adventures that lie in wait for early morning walkers.

I'm persuaded that the joys of walking begin with an open and curious mind, and a conscious sensitivity to sights, sounds and smells.

About walking in general Henry David Thoreau wrote *". . . YOUR MORALE IMPROVES; YOU BECOME FRANK AND CORDIAL, HOSPITABLE AND SINGLEMINDED."*

To those who already saunter, to those thinking of walking, to those who walk aerobically, to those who vigorously swing their arms or carry weights, to those who clamp on a headset to study or otherwise be entertained en route, to those who walk from here to there and back, to those who very deliberately walk only for their health, this book is dedicated to opening up new and rewarding experiences en route.

Echo and I hope you enjoy these tales before breakfast.

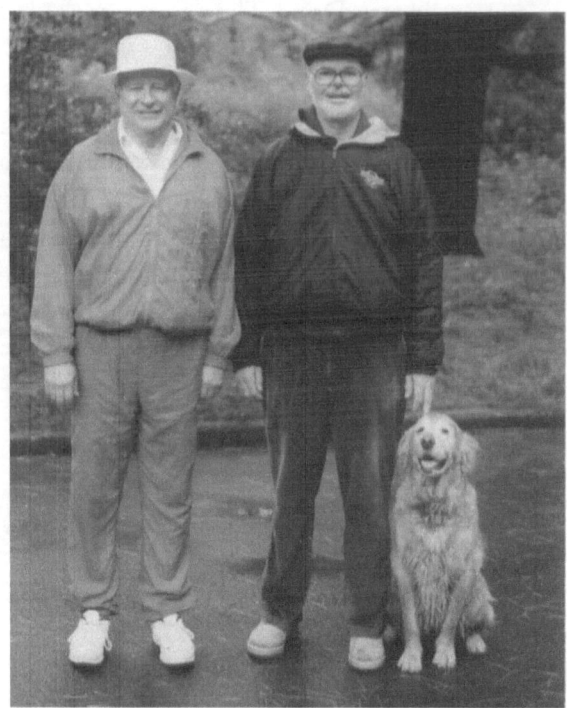

Gordon Fuqua
re-joins Herb
and Echo on
May 11, 1996
for 5000th
pre-breakfast
walk.

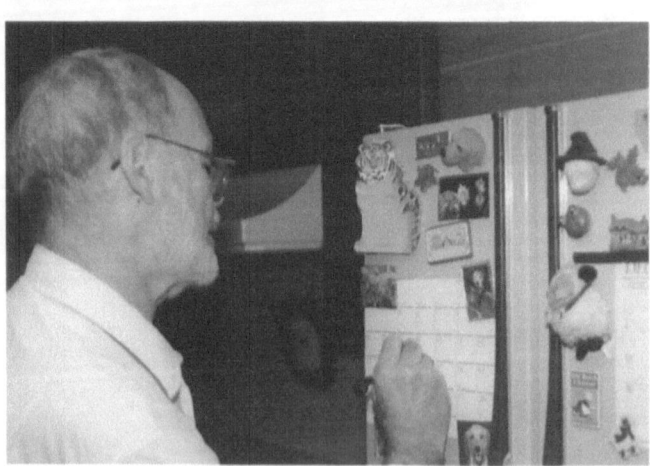

Posting mileage after every morning walk.

PREFACE

READY, GET SET AND WALK

"Few people know how to take a walk. The qualifications . . . are endurance, plain clothes, old shoes, an eye for nature, good humor, vast curiosity, good speech, good silence and nothing too much."

—Ralph Waldo Emerson

This book is about some of the thousands of walks I've enjoyed all over the world. While it is not a how-to book, before sharing more of my tales I thought I'd pass on some ideas on my how's and why's of walking.

First, the most important step for walking is a comfortable pair of shoes. There's extra spring, extra comfort in jogging or walking shoes available at any local athletic shoe store. Investing $40 or $70 makes all the difference in the world. Try several different models—walking or jogging shoes—either kind. Indeed, if you're not even sure you want to try walking, visit a shoe store and walk a few yards in a pair of walking shoes. The extra lift will convince you to start walking.

Second, dress comfortably for whatever is out there—cold, heat, rain, snow. So that you never have to think about what to wear, set aside your shoes, athletic socks, and walking clothes in an extra bathroom, or bedroom, or if you live in a warm climate, perhaps in the garage. In this way everything is organized and waiting in one spot. (On trips, if there is no room in a suitcase for walking basics, take along a small athletic bag.) To simplify walking in rainy weather, keep some walking boots or an old pair of walking shoes in a pair of rubbers or so you don't have to struggle to put them on. Bad weather boots, overcoats, scarves, umbrellas (have a big one handy) should be in your front or back hall closet as needed. Always wear a cap or hat in cold or cool weather to conserve body heat.

Third—and most important after comfortable walking shoes—is a pencil and pocket-size note pad or a piece of paper. It will retain a treasure trove of captured thoughts, plans for the day, reminders for this and that. Henry David Thoreau walked to exercise both his body and his mind, and Dr. Othneil J. Seiden, in his book "Walk! Get Into Shape the Easy Way" said it clearly:

"You will learn to control your creative abilities to work for you often while walking. Walking can actually unleash the genius in you!"

And, more on creativity during a walk, George Sheehan, *Philosopher of Fitness* article, "The Walking Magazine" wrote:

"Almost all the great thinkers who gave us the best books wrote them on their walks . . . If you're a walker you can put it all together. During the time you're walking, you can be thinking. The road becomes a gymnasium, a classroom, a cathedral—whatever you want."

Drink a glass of water with a little lemon juice and start walking. No need to warm up—that first easy fifty yards is all that is needed. Walking is its own warm-up. And never forget a pencil and pad to capture those thoughts and plans for the day!

How Far is a Walk?

Time, physical capability, and desire is how far a walk is. If you simply can't face the before-breakfast walk, time can be scheduled before lunch or dinner, or in the evening. However, if you want to walk every day there likely will always be inconveniences to disrupt whatever good intentions you may have—except before breakfast.

Once I had a 7 A.M. flight from Newark Airport. That meant leaving home at 5:30 and getting up by 5:00. So, why not get up at 4:30 and walk a few miles? Nugget and I went out into 25 degree weather with a full moon overhead. Not a car was on the road as my flashlight helped me keep an eye on Nugget. Then, thanks to adjusting to the spectacular moonlight, no flashlight was needed. The walk turned out to be one of the quietest and most serene walks I ever had. I was raring to go by the time I got to the airport.

How-to-walk books and medical articles suggest 3 to 4 half hour walks per week. To each his or her own. What is most important is disciplining one's self to a routine. As for your physical capability, start out easy and work up to your time limitations and physical needs and goals. One hundred yards out and back may be a limit for one person, five to six miles for another. While this book is not about walking for your health (a wonderful by-product, nonetheless), for those who are strictly health conscious and want to walk vigorously or aerobically, you and your doctor are likely the best judges of any physical limitations.

For the saunterer, desire is how far a walk is.

Nature's Aid

Almost 2500 years ago, Hippocrates said, *"WALKING IS MAN'S BEST MEDICINE."*

Today numerous surveys indicate walking is America's favorite form of exercise. It's more popular than jogging, or swimming, tennis, or golf. Walking burns just as many calories as jogging. It merely takes longer to walk the same distance. And, chances are when an easy paced walk ends you'll feel so good you'll want to go further.

Rebecca Hughes in Family Circle, May 1986 said

"Walking can help ward off depression, boost your energy level and help you to sleep more soundly. The reason behind these pleasant effects is a set of mood-elevating chemicals called endorphins, the body's natural opiates . . . endorphins help you feel refreshed and energized."

A Nike article in "Walk Nike" notes:

"Walking reduces headaches and tension, it sharpens the senses, it increases alertness, relieves depression and helps you feel younger. Unlike swimming, its a weight-bearing exercise. It stimulates new bone tissue growth so that old bone can actually regenerate and become less brittle, reversing the aging process. Walking makes you smarter. It increases glucose to your brain so you can think more systematically, improving your ability to solve problems. And, finally, walking is practically injury free. It's the one exercise you can use throughout life."

It's well known that walking can help prevent heart attacks and stroke by strengthening the heart, reducing cholesterol, and lowering blood pressure. Finally regular walkers are more successful in losing weight and usually can better maintain weight control.

How Fast A Walk?

Jane Brody in a "Personal Health" article in the New York Times, March 14, 1991 notes:

"adding to the confusion are the myriad names given to different walking styles: race walking, pace walking, fitness walking, aerobic walking, power walking, rhythmic walking, treadmill walking and mall walking, among others. Surely there can't be that many ways to put one foot in front of the other."

Walking for me is really none of the above. I walk at whatever pace is comfortable. I walk to ENJOY my outing. I seem to walk a bit slower when it's hot, more briskly when it's cold. Still my walks usually move along at enough of a pace to come back with a bit of a sweat.

The walker who comes home and wishes he had more time to walk another mile or two is someone who mentally and physically feels good. When a walker looks forward to a walk with keen anticipation—similar to the eagerness of a 12-year-old about to have an ice cream cone—when it's no longer "I must walk because it's good for my health," distance no longer becomes a concern. Such walkers are obviously stimulating both mind and body. Finally, the walker who sees a short cut and takes a long cut, is a walker for whom the joys of walking has taken hold.

Walking while away from home is always an adventure. Many times I have enjoyed early morning walks around Washington, D.C. past the grandeur of the White House, the Lincoln and the Jefferson Memorial, and the Smithsonian. 2500 miles northwest was the walk from my motel at the edge of town a mile into the city of Fargo, North Dakota. Few houses there were large, streets were wide and clean, and people smiled and said hello to me in this great American midwestern city. I've enjoyed early morning walks along the San Francisco waterfront, around the beautiful New England Dartmouth campus in Hanover, New Hampshire, through the residential section of Cheshire, Connecticut while visiting my daughter Mary and her family, from the top of a hill in Los Angeles down to the bottom near the Occidental College campus when visiting my cousin Burns Lee. (Finding my way back up those constantly intersecting winding hilly L.A. roads was a challenge.) As I age, I may forget names or dates but every walk away from home remains distinctly clear in my memory.

What To Take Along

Back home I seldom have identification with me. If I stumble or have an accident, I've concluded they will identify me quickly if I am taken to a local hospital.

However, no one knows me when I'm away from home. Before I venture out, I do several things:

I write my name on a piece of paper along with the address where I am staying, date it, and put it in my pocket.

I take a pad or piece of paper with a pen or pencil for possible notes.

If I am staying at a hotel, I take along the key to my room, some hotel matches, and write my name on a piece of paper.

I always take some money with me but seldom take a wallet.

As soon as I leave my overnight accommodations, I look at the nearby intersecting streets, and write down the street names of the streets.

With these simple preparations, I am ready for accidents or getting lost, with one exception. If I am in a non-English speaking city abroad, Bon Jour, "Nehi," or Gut Morgen isn't enough to talk my way back if I stray. I am particularly careful, therefore, to take hotel matches or some identification to show to a non-English speaking local to help me head back to my hotel.

How far afield to walk?

I am perhaps more venturesome than most. But, I don't walk down dark alleys or go in empty warehouses. Still,some of my best morning adventures have happened in cities and countrysides by venturing a goodly distance away from my starting point. In sixteen years of daily walking there probably have been 400 days of walking away from home. Most have been in unfamiliar territory making possible a new and different walking adventure each time. And that, of course, is what this book is all about.

I decided early on that always walking the same route could become monotonous. As in life itself, variety, however minor the change, can keep a daily walk interesting. What I haven't tried while walking is listening to an educational book or entertainment cassette to pass the time. Not only do I believe blocking out external sound can be dangerous (such as missing the sound of cars) but for me headsets block out nature's and man-made sounds that add to the pleasure of walking.

Reaching for a way to encourage elderly people to walk, a retired Army Colonel once suggested counting steps as a way to pass the time. Surely there are more creative and stimulating ways to walk so as to enjoy the sky, or birds, or flowers, or buildings, or encounters with old and new friends.

Wearing a pedometer not only tracks your mileage relatively accurately, it can be used to estimate distance from point A to point B. (A good pedometer costs $18 to $20. It's easily adjustable to your approximate stride and likely will be accurate within 10%.)

Walking Diversions

Bored while walking? Sing inside to yourself. Sing out loud. Forget some words? Hum in between. Smile at passers-by (and likely get a smile in return).

Footprints in the sand, or snow, or damp grass can provide a fun challenge. See if you can walk in somebody else's footprints—imagine who they might be—and where they were going.

Listen to the birds. Consciously tune out all extraneous noises and focus just on the birds. Stop and listen to the sound of distant trains.

Tuck in your tummy and hold it tight for 50 steps, then 75, then 100 steps. Flex your arm muscles and keep them tight for a minute. Who knows, maybe you can pull in your belt another notch next month.

Take along a tennis ball to squeeze and strengthen your hands. If you have your dog along toss a ball for retrieval.

Want to get aerobic? Go ahead and swing your arms up and down, or left and right. Within your limits, pick up your pace for a 100 yards or half a mile. You may come back perspiring and feel even better.

Are you steady on your feet? Find a large flat area—a level football field, a broad beach or a large empty parking lot and close your eyes. See if you can walk 25 or 50 paces in a straight line—as a blind person does. Then appreciate how sure-footed a blind person has to become.

Still, walking for me needs no such continued diversions. As my route may wander, so does my mind. Simply enjoying the dawn of a new day with its beauty or stormy elements or new scenery transcends the need for any artificial distractions.

How About Walking Companions?

Perhaps the best companion is a trained dog. He or she quietly loves you, doesn't intrude on your thoughts, sets you up to meet other people through other people's dogs, and may provide you an extra sense of security. An untrained dog—the one that pulls the master this way and that—can be a poor companion.

My 12-year-old companion Nugget, who grew old and tired, and Echo who followed her, have been the best companions a walking man could ever have. From the moment Echo wakes me, through her romps in the fields, the park, or on the golf course, until she returns often exhausted or wet from morning dampness or inclement weather, obedience-trained Echo is a joy of walking. Nugget and Echo have shared most of my walks—as you will see in succeeding chapters.

A spouse or friend can be a plus or minus on a walk: a plus for the joy of companionship and shared conversation, or a minus because the intrusion of conversation will likely be at the expense of wondrous thoughts, meditation or communing with nature. Frequently two fast walking constantly chattering walkers pass me during my morning walks. I cannot believe they see or hear any of the wonders around them.

Robert Louis Stevenson said it all:

"A walking tour should be gone upon alone because freedom is of the essence; because you should be able to stop and go on, and follow this way or that, as the trek takes you; and because you must have your own pace, and neither trot alongside a champion walker, nor mince in time with a girl. And then you must open to all impressions, and let your thoughts take colour from what you see . . . I want to see my vague notions float like the down of the thistle before the breeze, and not to have them entangled in the briars and thorns of controversy. For once, I like to have it all my way; and this is impossible unless you are alone."

CHAPTER 1

NO EXCUSES

"One of the pleasures of standing in a gentle snowstorm and watching flakes drift slowly earthward is the muffling quiet that envelops you like a second coat. The snowfall seems to absorb the noise of the world and a soft silence piles up all around."

—John Grossmann,
Listen to the Sounds of Silence,
"Creative Living," Winter 1989.

Nothing Needs To Stand In The Way Of A Walk

For those in generally good health there is never a reason to miss walking every day. All that is needed to become a never-fail early morning walker is to sample the glory of a few sunrises, stand in awe of beautiful clear skies, meet an old friend or make a new one, savor the smell of fresh baking or pretend to be a kid again in the rain or snow and inhale early morning air that is always crisper, fresher, and cooler than later in the day. Bad weather, rain and snow storms are the best excuses in the world to bundle up, take a walk, and be a kid again. What child did not revel stomping and splashing in the rain or inhaling the beauty and fun of snow?

From the edge of the bed Nugget poked her face into mine. Smiling from both ends, she was telling me it was time to get up and walk. It was a winter Saturday and I had looked forward to walking an easy mile to the Baptist Church to have waffles at their annual benefit. Unexpectedly during the night a heavy snow had fallen and now the world outside was white.

In the guest bathroom, I put on my cold weather red flannel long-johns, sweat pants and Princeton orange sweat jacket. As I sat putting on my bad weather boots, Nugget nuzzled me and wagged her tail eagerly. It was our daily routine.

From the front hall closet, I wrapped a scarf around my neck, put on my rabbit fur hat with ear flaps, stuck my arms into my waist level winter jacket in which I kept my gloves, drank my regular lemon juice-flavored warm glass of water, got Nugget's leash, and headed out the back door. I was prepared for the worst.

Nugget darted out and plunged into the 14-inch deep snow emerging with a white snowy snout. Both of us floundered—she with arching leaps, I with slow, short steps. I tossed a fluffy snowball in Nugget's face to watch her react playfully.

The roads were not yet plowed and with not a car in sight we lurched through the snow down the middle of Mercer Street. A marvelous after-snow quiet punctuated the beauty of our white winter wonderland. Today could not be a saunter. It was going to be a physical effort making that mile walk to town. Twenty-five minutes later, huffing and puffing, we walked down Nassau Street through the ruts left by a few cars, then down Chambers Street to the side door of the black Baptist Church. After tying up Nugget near the entrance I became the first and only customer for their annual $3.50 waffle breakfast. I ordered a second breakfast and gave Nugget half a waffle and a sausage. She voraciously gulped her reward. Among the black hosts were several familiar faces who had arrived early to decorate the church. As we prepared to leave a half hour later, only three more customers had arrived. Sensing the benefit was not going to be a success because of the heavy snow, I wrote a supplemental check since the benefit was for Ed Smith, the church minister, and a fellow Rotarian. He was going blind and needed help.

Back home an hour and a half after we started, Nugget shook off the snow that covered her from head to tail, and I had my usual after-walk glass of water. Except for my commitment to walking every morning before breakfast, I never would have had such a vigorous walk, nor had such a tasty breakfast, nor experienced such an unexpected good feeling in support of a good cause.

"People who walk only when the weather is fine and mild do not know what they miss. They deprive themselves of the enchantment of mist and fog, the soft splash of rain, the velvet touch of snow, the wild challenge of cold and wind, and languor of summer heat."

Aaron Sussman and Ruth Goode, "The Magic of Walking"

The rain was pounding on the roof when I arose at 6:15 am one morning in the little English village of Lyme Regis in Dorset. I put rubbers over my walking shoes, covered my jacket with a raincoat and, carrying an umbrella, headed down the hill towards the water. The wind turned my umbrella inside out which I was able to reverse as a small dock came into sight with several fishing dories tied up along side.

Fisherman's nets that had been stretched out to dry were now saturated. Carefully coiled ropes were swollen from the rain. Forlorn looking gulls overhead floated motionless as they headed into the strong wind. Stark, rainy, and desolate—it was the stuff of a Winslow Homer seascape. I stood on the dock, back to the wind and rain, inhaling fisherman smells of dead fish, oil and grease. A moment later, while fruitlessly searching the littered rocky beach for relics, a strong smell of kelp and seaweed completed the seaside aromas. I was a young boy again sloshing my way through an intriguing seaside adventure.

On the way back up the hill to the rundown 19th century wood and stucco Three Cups Hotel, I found a novelty store where I purchased stamps and postcards and tucked a London paper under my arm inside my raincoat. A few moments later I arrived at the hotel sopping wet from the knees down, chilled after 45 minutes in the storm, and ready for a warm shower. At breakfast my wife and my 90 year old mother were subjected to a step-by-step report on my Lyme Regis morning outing. I sensed by their indulgence they thought me a bit unhinged. But for me, I had a memorable, exciting adventure walk.

It was very much like a description by Harrison E. Salisbury in *The Good Health Magazine* article from "The New York Times Magazine," April 16, 1989:

"To be certain, the world-class place to walk on the beach in the rain is Nauset Beach on Cape Cod, the rain slanting in, the gray sea boiling, the breakers crashing, the smell of kelp and brine, oilskins yellow and flapping, water streaming down your face, great gusts of oxygen hurling into your lungs, wild

flights of cream-and-dun gulls, the air singing with salt, the sand firm and live under your feet. Roaring a chantey at the top of your lungs and not hearing a word of it. No excitement like it."

After particularly heavy rains, Princeton's Stony Brook overflows and covers Quaker Road. I had heard the heavy rain all night and wondered if the police would close the road. Sure enough, the next morning the road was barricaded permitting Echo and me to walk down the middle of what normally is a busy commuter road. A mile down the road we were at the edge of a temporary lake covering the road and fields on either side. The surging water, carrying along massive debris, was five to six feet above normal stream level. Low limbs of trees now in mid stream were bending against the water. Echo walked into the new lake, dog paddled this way and that, came out and shook hard. To the east a faint glow suggested the rain clouds would soon be passing. Returning to the road barrier, two cars and their frustrated drivers were turning around. I knew the road would be re-opened in a few hours when the waters receded. I'd enjoyed this walk before and knew it was only a question of time and elements before Echo and I could plan to have the road to ourselves again.

Long ago I dismissed bad weather, aches, pains, bronchitis, colds, tiredness, and late hours the night before as excuses not to walk. Once, after spending the night under observation in the Special Care section of the hospital for a false-alarm heart condition, I got up early and walked around the corridors. A nurse spotted me with "What *ARE* you doing, Mr. Hobler? Get right back in bed! People on this floor simply don't do things like that." Happily, I'd already walked my mile and checked out an hour later.

One afternoon I stepped off a curb, inadvertently twisted my ankle, and suffered a severe sprain. After a restless night, I woke up to consider my consecutive morning walking streak might end after 2465 days.

Gingerly putting my injured foot on the floor by my bed, I took one step and quickly pulled my leg back up. Getting from the bedroom down the hall to the guest bathroom was agony. I eased a slipper on my swollen right foot as Nugget nuzzled me, put on my left walking shoe, and limped through the house in great pain. It was one slow, painful step at a time to the back door. Was it possible to make it to the end of the driveway? Several times I stopped and considered returning. Step by agonizing step I went—10 yards—50 yards—100 yards. Half way up the street I was adjusting to the pain. 3 miles later it was gone! And that effort, along with hundreds of others, provides me with one more walking memory.

I realized that day there are many people who are permanently or temporarily incapacitated for whom walking is a real effort. Each determined step for them may be a victory. Until that day when I may be totally incapacitated by hospitalization or serious illness, there will be no excuses for me not to walk every morning for each walk provides a mental, physical and spiritual uplift with daily thankfulness for being able to enjoy the wonderment of life.

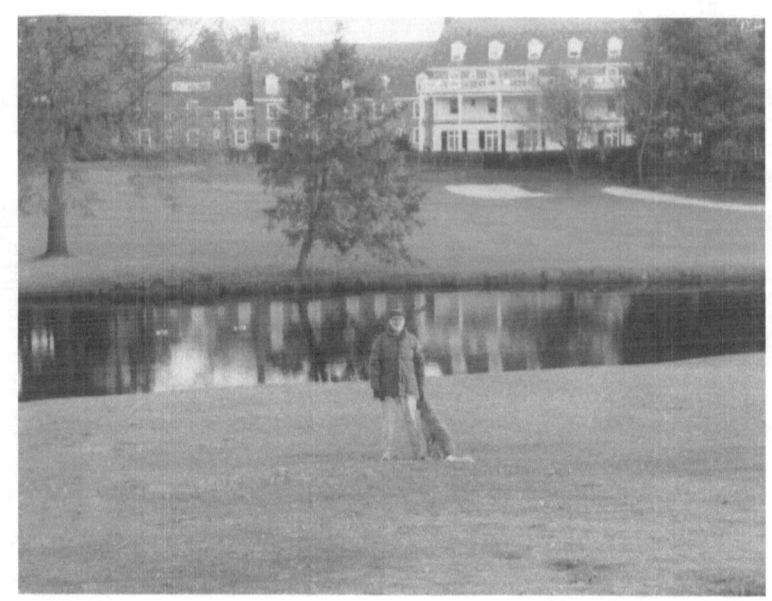

3000th consecutive morning, November 20, 1990 in Princeton.

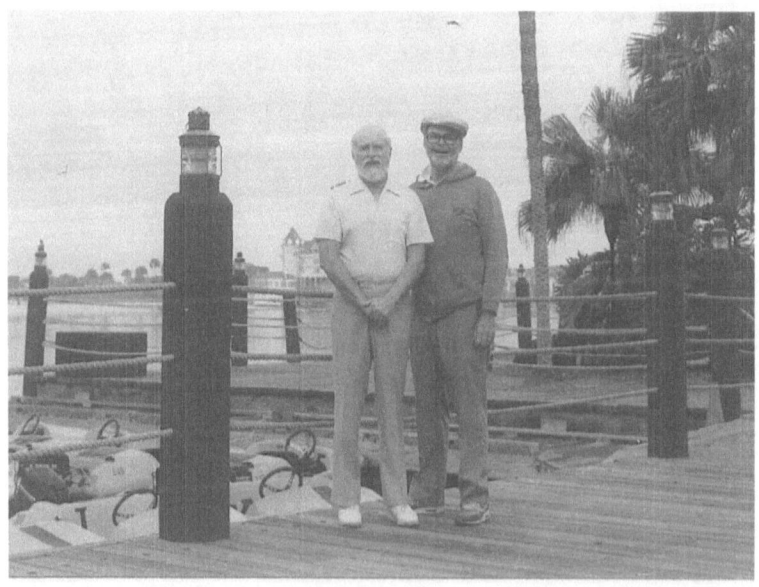

2000th consecutive morning, Disney World, Florida. February 14, 1988 with Gordon Fuqua who started me walking.

CHAPTER 2

RIGHT AROUND HOME

"Once I've set out, I discipline myself to avoid all direct routes of any kind, to reject any sense of purpose, or progress, to resist all temptations to accomplish anything of foreseeable use. My sole aim is to be diverted from my path; to be caught by the first crocus or to loiter beside a stray daffodil."

Robert Finch, *Crossing Paths*, "The Walking Magazine," April/May 1987

For me, constantly walking from here to there and back is no fun. It invariably becomes monotonous, uninspiring and leads to few new experiences.

Looking for a different way to walk each day is the beginning of walking for the joy of walking. Starting from my doorstep there are hundreds of different walking routes.

For example: From my driveway on Mercer Road I can turn left or right. If I turn left, after one block I can go straight, turn left or turn right–three choices of direction. One block later I'll have another three choices–and so on.

With a little planning there are dozens of different routes in the immediate area that make walking an adventure. For variety tomorrow reverse today's route. Going beyond the immediate neighborhood opens up hundreds of different route combinations that can provide a new world of walking experiences.

Whether in the country or city, you'll likely have to walk on roads from time-to-time. It's best to walk against traffic so you can take evasive action if necessary. If, as I have sometimes done, you are creatively thinking about something, bring your mind back into focus before you cross a road.

At least twice in my many years of walking I awakened from my walking reverie just in time.

There is no question that the regularity of my regular morning walks has come from the stimulation of seeking different routes while keeping my eyes and mind open to enjoy whatever comes along. Chances are that wherever you live—in center city, in suburban towns, or in the open space of country villages—there are many paths to provide variety in walking.

In Einstein's Footsteps

Shortly after the start of my early morning walks I "discovered" the Institute for Advanced Study woods just down the road a few hundred yards. Previously, I never had an occasion to walk in this almost pristine woods through which people like Einstein and Oppenheimer—and our growing-up children—had once walked. Wandering through the 600 acres of woods, crossing over its streams, and along the Delaware Raritan Canal, suddenly I felt was a thousand miles away from civilization.

After four or five walks through the woods on many trails, I decided to try to plot them. How many were they? How far from this one to the next? What was the total mileage of all of the trails put together? Had anyone ever thought to make a booklet showing the paths to encourage walkers to explore every part of the woods?

Using my pedometer for measurements, I returned day after day to draw a map of the 15 or more trails I discovered. I began to feel like an early American pioneer laying out a map of uncharted frontiers.

Nugget was always finding narrow new paths branching out from the main path that offered new exploring opportunities for us both. Day after day, I returned to further explore and measure each new trail.

Frequently deer bounced through the underbrush. One day I tip-toed past two men with binoculars studying birds in the trees. Another morning I spotted a young couple on the ground in their sleeping bag and on another, a young couple was having breakfast along side the canal.

Over several months I walked and re-walked the wooded trails checking and rechecking my distances. One day with great pride I walked into the administration office of the Institute of Advanced Study holding my completed map in hand.

"May I help you?" the receptionist asked.

"Yes," I said, "My name is Herb Hobler and I live over on Mercer Street. I walk each morning and in the last several months have walked all over your beautiful woods charting each and every path. They total 8.2 miles. I thought perhaps you would like to have a copy of my trail map to reproduce it for others."

Smiling graciously she said, "Oh, Mr. Hobler. We are so grateful for your thoughtfulness and efforts. We are most appreciative. Perhaps you would like this little guide we have already put together."

I compared their map to the one I had diligently and carefully recorded. It was an almost exact duplicate of every curve, distance and intersection I had laid out. Fortunately I did not know about their trail map earlier, for my morning explorations had been a far better adventure without following a map.

****

It was an early spring Sunday morning as Nuggett and I rounded historical Nassau Hall on the university campus where the Continental Congress met in 1783. There, just below the bell tower, were 10 to 12 men bowling black balls about the size of a softball. One man would roll his ball 20-25 yards and, after it came to a dead stop, another man would roll his black ball to try and hit it.

The men, most of whom looked over 60, had swarthy complexions and definitely were not dressed for church.

"What kind of game is this?" I asked.

"Itsa calleda Bocce" responded one man. "Itsa an olda Italiano game. We beena playeda hera twice a month fora years."

As I watched the game, better understanding how a second or third player would gain point position by knocking balls off the course, one younger man commented:

"Many of these men are immigrants, but Dad came over from Italy about 1910 and he used to play this game with other university employees way back then." It was then I recalled how many Italian immigrants had helped build university dormitories in the 1920's and 30's. There was something very special watching the fellowship and spirit of these men playing their native Italian sport on the campus they helped to build. It was an unexpected and rewarding fifteen minute interlude in my walk.

****

Princeton University's athletes and campus facilities have provided many unexpected early morning pleasures. One fall morning at 7:30 I came upon the 150 pound football team practicing. Another day the girls field hockey team was about to leave by bus. Almost any early morning the various men and women's crews are out practicing on Lake Carnegie. Saturday mornings in the winter at 7 am dozens of 8-10 year-olds are playing Pee Wee Hockey at Baker Rink.

Jadwin Gym is an extraordinary sports complex. On the below-ground level is a huge dirt floor large enough for the football and baseball teams to practice in inclement weather. Eight tennis courts are on the same floor. In floors above are squash courts and training rooms while on the upper floor is a huge area housing the basketball court and stands for 7000 fans. A few feet from the court is a complete indoor track facility.

Nugget trotted along side me one Sunday morning when I veered off my usual route to walk to the back side of this huge building. Cars were parked up and down the hill and in the parking lot beyond. What possibly could be happening at 7:30 am on a Sunday morning at Jadwin? Certainly it wasn't a basketball game or squash tournament.

A large basement doorway was open, large enough to drive in a big truck. I stepped inside to see a totally unexpected sight of young women in horse show regalia riding their horses around the outside perimeter of the dirt floor. I climbed up some steps so as to look down on the scene of perhaps 30 horses and riders warming up for a horse show. Around and around they trotted as maintenance men moved different hurdles into place. After watching for ten minutes, Nugget strained at her leash watching the horses so we departed so as not to disturb them. My decision to alter my route and explore the rear of the building had provided me an unexpected and pleasurable experience.

One Saturday morning a big bus was parked by the the dressing rooms adjoining Jadwin Gym and Palmer Stadium. Crowded around it was the whole Princeton football team loading up their gear for a trip to New Haven to play Princeton's traditional rival. At 7 am few students or fans were on hand to send them off.

"How are they going to do today against Yale, Coach?" I asked.

It had been 11 years since Princeton had beaten their arch rival. "THIS year we're out to beat them" he replied.

I watched them get on board, gave them a "V" for victory sign, and a "yea, Tigers" cheer. That afternoon I listened to the game on the radio feeling a special kinship with the players for having mixed with them early that morning. My cheering didn't help. The Bulldogs beat the Tigers for the 12th year in a row.

Again, this time on an early spring day about 7:30, I walked past the head of the football stadium and noticed the main gate was open. Just inside were dozens of men with bicycles.

"What are you all doing here at this time of morning?" I asked.

"This is the starting point of our bike rally" replied a man about 30 years old. Like most of the others, he was attired in skintight black clothing similar to a wet suit. It showed off his trim muscular body.

Sheepishly I asked, "What's a bike rally?"

"We are divided into several groups by age and ability. Starting from here, they have mapped out routes covering from 30 to 75 miles all over this part of New Jersey. Some riders will return here after a few hours, some after 5 or 6 hours."

He showed me a map for his 50 mile race. A thermos containing water was strapped to his bike. Unlike the horizontal bars of bikes in my day that let you sit up straight, all these racing bikes had inverted grips. My back ached watching them crouch over the bars.

To send off the first 15 or 20 riders a judge called out some instructions and fired a starting gun. Nugget flinched, the cyclists made a hasty departure, and we moved on from our unexpected walking highlight.

Cemeteries may not be a good place to take up permanent residence, but they are fascinating places to visit. I paused in front of a Princeton cemetery headstone. "William Windsor departed this life age 97." Who was he, what did he accomplish in his lifetime? Would that headstones told more about those resting below.

Nearby was a large family monument with 8 small horizontal stones. There obviously was room for more stones in the years to come. Twenty feet away "God Bless Baby Alice" recorded an obvious tragedy for some young couple. Nearby were four monoliths with Chinese inscriptions. Then I spotted old friend Nat McKee's headstone with its affectionate tribute "To Pop Pop from his grandchildren."

I stopped for a moment in the President's section. Many of the university presidents are buried there including Aaron Burr. No need to stop by and say hello again to Grover Cleveland and his obelisk. I'd done that many times. He lived and died in Princeton after his Presidency. (A half mile from my house in the sometimes visited Quaker Cemetery is the headstone of Richard Stockton, a signer of the Declaration of Independence.) It is always impressive to stand by the headstones of these great men and consider their roles in our American heritage.

Exploring further, I found some familiar names in the northwestern section. One, a recent grave with a temporary marker, identified Paul Hinds. What a wonderful, kind gentleman Paul had been. For 35 years or more he had faithfully come by our house each week to cart away trash. At the start Paul had charged only $2.00 per week. A short, thin man, he always had a smile, always spoke softly. He was a special, lovely man.

Close by was the headstone of another black friend and then another. During my undergraduate days at Princeton I was involved with many black youngsters through YMCA work. Later as a resident I served on an Interracial Housing board and on various inter-racial committees. In the 18th and 19th centuries this section of the cemetery had been set aside exclusively for Negroes. Now blacks and all races and creeds are located throughout the cemetery.

There were no headstones in the new northeastern corner of the cemetery but two small temporary markers caught my attention. I stooped over to instantly recognize the names of Kitty and Jose Menendez, recent residents of Princeton who were murdered while they were in Los Angeles the year before. Their sons, one a Princeton student, had been indicted for the murder. The story made national news services.

I always stop by our family granite monument with the hickory marker engraving "Virginia Hobler Redpath, August 10, 1920-December 26, 1947." My sister had died a month after giving birth to a girl. Next to her was my father "Atherton W. Hobler September 2, 1890-January 3, 1974." The most recent stone—which had been partially inscribed with a name and birth date at the same time my father died—was now finally marked: "Ruth Windsor Hobler June 13, 1893-May 23, 1989." Twenty of us had gathered around my mother's marker in sorrow and in celebration for her great spirit. My two brothers and I had lowered her ashes into the ground. This grand lady had left 20 grandchildren and 21 great-grands. Next to her was another granite marker, "Our friend Jessie Johns." Jessie had been the closest thing to a Nanny any of our children ever had. An old friend of my mother, she had become a part of the family moving from family to family as new babies were born. Upon her death no one in her own family wished to claim her remains. My practical mother kept her ashes in a closet for over a year, and then lovingly decided to bury her in our family plot.

One Saturday morning Nugget and I took one of our long weekend walks across town and passed by a white framed house on Princeton Avenue. Graham Rohrer and I had commuted for years to New York on the old Pennsy railroad. His newspaper was on the sidewalk. Taking out my notepad, I wrote a note, signed it "Herbie, your morning delivery boy," stuck it inside the paper, and put the paper on his front stoop. A few weeks later we met up town and he said,

"Herbie, your delivery service isn't very regular. I've had to go out to the street every day since you dropped by. It's very irritating!"

His comment so tickled me that thereafter every few weeks I'd go out of my way to pass his home, write another note, and place the paper on his stoop. One morning he caught me in the act and, with a big smile, invited me in. I'd already walked my minimum mile before breakfast so while Nugget waited patiently outdoors I enjoyed a light breakfast interlude with Graham and Jane before heading on home.

Fred's grandfather lived nearby beyond the intersection of Bayard Lane and Route 206. Driving to visit him one very warm afternoon, Fred came to the intersection and stopped behind a car. The car ahead decided to take an impermissible right turn at the red light. Thus thinking the light had changed, Fred moved forward to cross the road. A large truck waiting to turn left into his road blocked the view of an on-coming car on the other side of the truck. His was an old car with no air conditioning so the windows were open and, sadly, he did not have on a seat-belt when the other car going 40 mph hit his car amidships. His car rolled over. Twenty-six year old Fred Woodbridge, outstanding involved citizen, stockbroker, night school law student, political activist, and son of close friends, was almost instantly killed in a one-in-a-million accident.

Some weeks later I crossed the intersection thinking about this tragic event and found small bits of glass at the accident site. There was a tape cassette by the curb, one obviously he had listened to in his car. I picked it up, put it in my pocket to later give to Polly and Dudley, the Godparents of one of our children and the bereaved parents of an exceptional young man.

My walks frequently take me through that intersection. The bits of glass have disappeared. The vivid memories of Fred remain.

Len Johnson had a keen sense of humor and was always handy with slightly off-color stories at our weekly Saturday lunch bunch. After a series of strokes he was moved from the hospital to Merwick Nursing Home near the YMCA. Even though he was not responsive in any way, some of us would stop in to visit. After tying up Echo outside, I would wander through the hallways past the ill and elderly to his room. Sometimes his eyes were open seeing nothing. "Hi, Len. This is Herb Hobler. I hope you can hear me. We are all thinking about you." No reaction even to holding his hand. Still, just in case he could hear inside his non-responsive body, I always felt there was special purpose to my morning walk to stop in and, perhaps, make my presence known to him.

A Walk Through My Town

"When you're feeling a little down, it wouldn't hurt to take a nice brisk walk around the neighborhood to help you feel better!"
—Sara E. Sondgrass, Asst. Professor of Psychology, Skidmore College as quoted in "Aerobic Walking for Fitness & Health"

Share with me a leisurely but wonderful example of how a one-hour walk can be so fulfilling.

The Princeton University campus provides dozens of different scenic and interesting routes. I had crossed over to Route 206, continued a mile up to Nassau Street, then on to the University campus, and down to the railroad station just in time to see retired Brigadier General George Eggers ready to board the train. After some banter, I went across campus past the tennis courts (the freshman baseball diamond in my time) and along a path past several dormitories towards Washington Road. Once this path had been a public road. The university had closed it to eliminate automobile traffic through the campus.

At the edge of Washington Road a backhoe was digging deep in the ground in what obviously was going to be a very large basement. "Going to be an extension of the bio building" said one of the workmen. Echo pulled back as the bucket reared up like the head of a huge dinosaur, spun around and dumped some dirt.

Past Isabella McCosh Infirmary we went, and through the gardens of Prospect (once the home of the college Presidents and now a faculty dining facility). Woodrow Wilson said goodbye to his university family there at the Porte co-chere when he went off to be President of the United States. It too had been his home as university president.

Near Prospect is the huge gothic university chapel similar in magnitude and style to many churches in England. Once the Christian center of what had been a Presbyterian founded college, it is now used by members of all faiths. I tied Echo to a post and entered the empty chapel to marvel at the magnificence of the structure to enjoy a few moments of meditation. A few minutes later Echo greeted me outside with that worried canine "where did you go" look. After untying her leash she took off out of sight through the archway of Chancellor Green. In the forties it had been the college library, then already an ancient building, and now a student center. Under the archway were stapled scores of student announcements. "Slightly beat up lounge chair—$15—452-6889," "Need a ride to Ft. Lauderdale April 10th. 258-4386," "Need fridge—CHEAP. Call after 10 pm 258-6689," "GALAP Meeting Tuesday, Murray Dodge, 8 pm" (Gay and Lesbian Association of Princeton), "Hot pizzas. Delivered to your room—24 hrs. a day. 924-0090."

Just beyond the bulletin board in an open air courtyard I stopped to recall an extraordinary experience one morning during a walk several years before. Three or four people had been standing perfectly still looking up into one of the trees. I had slowly edged forward to see a small bird that had been the focus of their attention. A moment later it flew off.

An obviously knowledgeable spectator had observed "It's a very rare bird that seldom has ever been seen in the United States. Its normal habitat is Costa Rica. We can't imagine how it could ever have come this far north. It's been roosting in that tree on and off for the last three days." The next day the local paper reported on the phenomenon and identified the bird, though the name has since escaped me.

Now Echo was out of sight and my whistle was for naught. Suddenly she came racing around Nassau Hall. This was but the first of many times thereafter that Echo made a game of racing behind a building only to reappear after having run completely around it.

We walked across the front campus, through the opened FitzRandolph Gate, which, until the student protests of 1969, was closed all year except on graduation day. Traffic at 8 am on Nassau Street was getting heavier as we waited for safe passage to walk across Princeton's main street to Palmer Square.

Should I stop by the Squires Choice and get one of those freshly baked banana walnut muffins? Should I start that diet today or get that muffin? The muffin won. To Palmer Square I went, dropped Echo's leash in a loop over a parking meter, bought the still warm muffin, and headed home to conclude my university stroll.

A house on the way home was for sale. Spread out on the lawn were household goods, furniture and paintings. Fellow Rotarian and real estate agent Jim Firestone stepped out the front door carrying a large box.

"What's going on here, Jim?" I inquired.

"This 1905 house is up for sale and we are holding an auction this afternoon for everything in the house not being passed on to the family members" he responded.

Jim then gave me a personal tour from top to bottom of the empty house. We passed by six vintage telephones, a beautiful old mantel piece, and out through an old fashioned kitchen. The house needed a thorough cleaning.

My one hour morning walk had been through familiar territory but with unexpected experiences: I had met an old friend, watched new construction, briefly meditated in the chapel, read some amusing student bulletins, heard a unique bird story, bought a muffin, and had a conducted tour of a large house for sale.

An open mind, an adventuresome outlook, and a bit of curiosity had converted what could have been just another 3 mile walk into a very special outing.

Nugget had no interest in chasing squirrels even when she was a young pup. On the other hand, Echo, her successor, chases after every one she sees. Usually there are four or five squirrels by Erdman Hall on the Theological Seminary campus on Library Place. Keeping Echo on leash, I tiptoe under an arch, moving slowly so as not to scare off any squirrels. Echo's ears go up as she slowly peers around the corner, her nose quivers and once she spots a squirrel she freezes. Occasionally a friendly squirrel will come within 8 to 10 feet. It is almost more than a restrained Echo can stand. She knows the route and I am sure anticipates the squirrel encounters. It's a highlight of that route for both of us.

One of the longest but most satisfying walks right around home was a regular Sunday morning walk five miles out into the country to have breakfast with my mother. Nugget was trained to be safely off leash all the way even as cars sped by a few feet from us. Echo, who succeeded Nugget when mother was 95, stayed on leash all the way. I just couldn't be sure of her if a squirrel or deer suddenly appeared.

I guess going home for some of Mom's cooking is something special for just about everyone. My mother would greet us at the door and give the dog a pat ("Yes I do love you, but I don't like your dog hairs in my living room"). She had the kitchen all ready for action. I'd always sit on the high stool near the stove as she cooked the eggs (the sausage was cooked and being kept warm), the coffee was perking, the jam was in place, and the toast was "popped" into the toaster. With the dog lying at our feet we'd spend 20 minutes or so eating side by side. ("Won't you have some more, dear?") Physically and mentally alert at her advanced age, she'd end breakfast with "I'll clean up later, dear" and then, with the dog in the back seat, I'd drive with her into town to buy her Sunday paper before returning to my house. While later a live-in companion would drive her, until she was 93 she'd take over and drive back home.

Those one-way walks to Mom's on Sunday morning were the best of all. And those five miles, mostly uphill, were always worth every single one of the 10,000 steps.

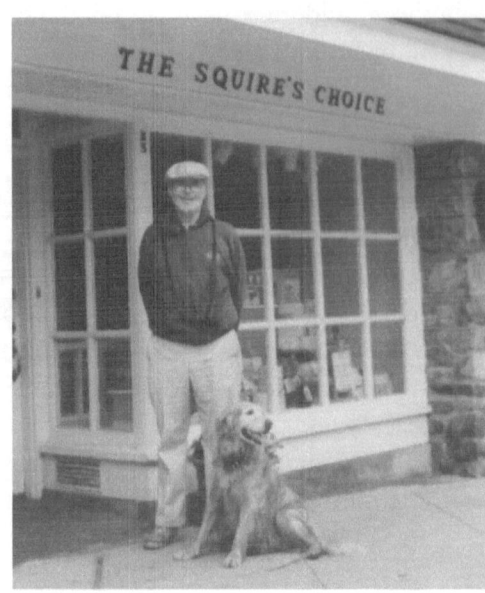

**A Walk
Around
Town:**
Stopping for
a fresh muffin
at 7 a.m.
Day 4999

Visiting
Nassau Hall on
the Princeton
University
campus
Day 4999

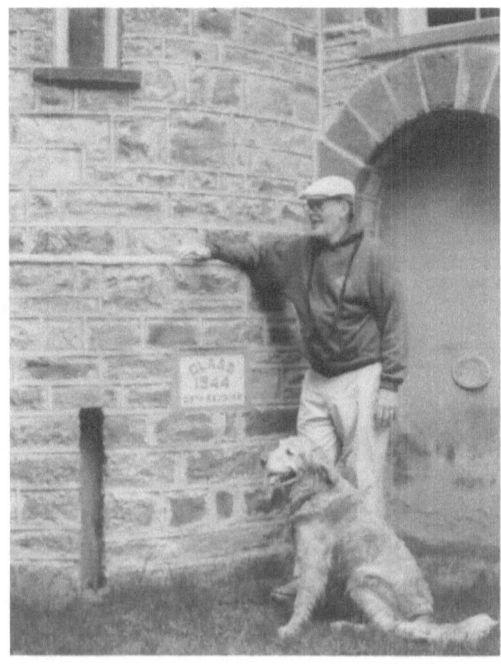

CHAPTER 3

LIFT YOUR SIGHTS

"Up there, alone with the wind and the sky and the steep grassy slopes, I nearly always find after a while that I am beginning to think more clearly . . . it is as if my mind, set free by space and solitude and oiled by the body's easy rhythm, swings open and releases thoughts it has already formulated."
—Colin Fletcher, "The Complete Walker III"

"Chin up!" my mother used to say when I seemed dejected. She knew what she was talking about. Certainly those who are caught up in their problems are more likely to look down. (And walkers ever mindful of where they are stepping don't look up enough.) But LOOKING UP lifts your spirits for there's a whole different world UP THERE above the pavement, curbs, sidewalks, and grass. All it takes is a little imagination and alert eyes, ears and noses.

Depending on the time of day and atmospheric conditions the sky UP there presents ever changing cloud murals of colors and shapes. The high, thin, whispish cirrus clouds of winter are frequently intermingled with airplane vapor trails. The misty, rainy looking nimbus clouds seemingly portend bad weather because they *LOOK* wet. In warm weather magnificent billowy cumulus clouds can look like faces, powder puffs, pillows, or marshmallows. Cloud shadows and colors created by the sun add magnificence to their ever changing patterns. The beauty of towering thunderheads is offset by the threat of impending lightning and storm.

The observant up-looking walker can absorb the beauty of, and fantasize all kinds of images from clouds that no artist could better conceive. Second to none is the glory of an absolutely clear blue sky at sunrise especially when, on an early cold winter morning, the moon has yet to be chased away by the sun.

UP there are soaring birds and squadrons of honking geese seasonally flying north or south. UP there is an occasional floating hot air balloon suddenly disturbing the quiet of the sky as its blast of flaming heat thrusts it higher in the air.

Closer to earth (but UP there) are flags waving, trees harboring a bird's nest, TV antennas on top of cable-less homes, houses and buildings with varieties of architectural styles. High up on Princeton University buildings in my home town are dozens of fascinating gargoyles I had never noticed before I looked UP.

UP there are chimneys of many sizes and shapes. In cold weather they spout smoke that spirals straight up into a windless sky or scatters aimlessly in the breeze. UP there is a church steeple reaching toward the heavens, a community landmark symbolizing peace and hope. Atop the steeple is a weather vane and just below is a catwalk around the church bell housing. Next door is a house with a gray asphalt shingled roof, across the street a slate roof next to one covered with rust-colored terra cotta. Leaves are sticking out of the gutters of one house, pine needles are lying on the roof of another. Houses along the street display a variety of square, standard, double hung, half moon, and picture windows. UP there is a gable with a small window. (Remember as a child looking through such an attic window from inside and fantasizing about the world below?)

Of all the looking up at houses during my morning walks the most memorable was in Castle Corfe, England. On the second floor of an open window, regally resting on the sill, was the snout of a Golden Retriever dog. The eyes in his immobile head followed my every movement. Sitting primly next to his head was a cat also looking down at me. It was such an extraordinary sight that I went back to my hotel and brought back my wife Randy and my camera to capture the sight. The cat and dog, obviously the best of friends, were still there. Little did we know that apparently we had happened upon a famous pair. Three years later in another part of England in a gift shop, we spotted a post card of this same dog and cat at the same window sill. It almost perfectly matched the captivating photo I had taken.

UP there are birds. One spring morning thousands of small birds erupted out of the woods and swirled up into the sky. It was an incredible, unexpected, unexplained explosion of birds. I watched in fascination for ten minutes until they disappeared. Near the same spot at Battlefield Park one cold November morning an old friend who had taken up walking after heart surgery came towards me. Suddenly we heard the honking of geese. Over the trees they came in formation by the hundreds. It was like a World War II armada of planes with one goose leading the pack. The leader turned north and the rest followed. Who decides to be the leader? How and why do they do that? We stood still to watch and listen to an extraordinary spectacle of nature. It was a shared moment we would talk about months later when next we met.

An uplifting walking experience can also come from looking DOWN. During my 6000 days of consecutive pre-breakfast walking I've found pennies, nickels, dimes, quarters, a five dollar bill, even a twenty dollar bill. My grandchildren's piggy banks have prospered.

It was 6:30 am. I was looking DOWN at the sidewalk on Nassau Street in Princeton. I spotted a credit card, picked it up, noted a woman's name, and when I got home I looked her up in the phone book. There she was—Anna Jones. I waited until 9 am to call. No, she hadn't lost it, her pocketbook had been stolen two days before in Trenton—10 miles away. The pocketbook had been returned to her by another person who had found it devoid of cash but still containing three of her four credit cards. She had been frantic about the missing card and was ebullient upon receiving my call.

"Would you like me to mail it to you?" I asked. "No," she responded, "What if it got lost again? Can I meet you somewhere? I work the night shift at the hospital, get off work about 7 am and I could meet you in front of the bank about 7:15 am."

And so we met early the next day, a Sunday, the only two people on the street. With both hands she gratefully grasped my hand containing the card and offered me $10, which I declined, and several days later she sent me a delightful thank-you letter. What a wonderful self-satisfying UP it was by looking DOWN.

Not every DOWN has to be an unexpected encounter. Ann had been very much a part of our community life and had a special interest in ecology. She was particularly interested in keeping our town neat and tidy. When she died of cancer, in her honor some friends announced an annual four day litter pick up throughout the town—organized block by block— to look DOWN and pick up trash from neighborhood streets. That first morning was a special experience for me as it must have been for the scores of other friends who had been provided a green trash bag. This day I must have stooped over 40 times. It was distressing to see the thoughtlessness of people who had dropped sandwich wrappers, a McDonald's bag, soft drink cans and beer bottles, used Kleenex, food wrappers, a rag, cigarette packages, a single glove, and candy wrappers. Twenty minutes later the green bag was almost filled, our neighborhood was neater and Ann had been remembered each time I had looked down. It was a lasting tribute for now frequently I pick up litter on the way home.

Perhaps my most interesting DOWN day was when I spotted a large X-ray film on the sidewalk. A few feet beyond was another—and then another. Feeling that I was invading someone's privacy, I held several of them up to the light. My laymen's diagnosis deduced that the first X-ray was that of a woman's chest. The second film was obviously of a skull. Fifty yards further I found a large brown envelope with two more X-rays and the address of a doctor in Hightstown, 10 miles away. I carefully put the 8 or 9 X-rays back in the brown envelope and returned home.

An hour later, I called the doctor's office to ask "Did you lose any X-rays?" Back came an excited and anxious female voice. "Oh, where did you find them? I had the envelope above the back seat of my convertible and didn't miss them until I got to work." The doctor's nurse had no idea where she had lost them and was effusively grateful for having them retrieved. I didn't ask for the diagnosis. But my downs that day gave me a very special upper.

CHAPTER 4

THE EARLY BIRD CATCHES THE SCENT

"Nothing is more memorable than a smell. One scent can be unexpected, momentary and fleeting, yet conjure up a childhood summer beside a lake in the mountains; another, a moonlit beach; a third, a family dinner of pot roast and sweet potatoes during a myrtle-mad August in a Midwestern town."
—Diane Ackerman, "A Natural History of the Senses"
(Random House)

There is a whole world of interesting smells to savor during early morning walks, many of which instantly recall pleasant memories. The smoke of a family fireplace or a Christmas tree, like the smell of freshly baked breads or frying bacon, brings back a feeling of childhood peace and security.

Encountering bakery smells have frequently stimulated my morning outlook, sharpened my appetite and enlarged my horizons about bakery products as far afield as London, Hong Kong, Beijing and Anchorage, Alaska. I encountered it first one winter morning about 7 A.M. as I walked by a specialty bakery in downtown Princeton called the Squires Choice. The aroma of fresh baking seeped through the front door. It was an overwhelming attraction and, since there were no signs prohibiting dogs, Nugget followed me into the store just as the baker was taking out a pan of steaming blueberry muffins. I picked out a hot one even as my olfactory senses encountered other smells of freshly ground coffee and cheeses. During my walk home the lingering aroma of my blueberry muffin escaping from the bakery bag continually whet my appetite. Nugget, whose nose began twitching with hungry anticipation, and who usually heeled close to my left knee, moved from my left to my right depending upon which hand was carrying the aromatic blueberry muffin.

I was strolling through a cobblestone square near the river front in Providence, Rhode Island. On a hill at the top of the square was a typical New England church with white clapboard siding and tall steeple. Below in the harbor was a multitude of boats including an old frigate reminiscent of early 19th century sailing ships. The square had perhaps a dozen 18th century style storefronts. My visual enjoyment of the scene was suddenly interrupted by a bakery aroma. I walked inside to see the baker in the process of making every conceivable goody including chocolate chip cookies. I'm ready for a warm chocolate chip cookie any time of day. Still, I'd never had a hot one at 7 A.M. so one promptly melted in my mouth as 3 more went back with me to my hotel to share later with my wife. That walk became a wonderful chocolate walking memory.

It was 6:45 and I already had walked around the exotic Bergen, Norway u-shaped harbor past a variety of schooners, scows, private yachts, small inboard and outboard boats, and a variety of fishing boats, a few of which had already returned with their early morning catch. I stood on the dock to watch an old salt toss fish accurately from the deck into a barrel on the dock. The deck of an adjoining boat was being hosed down while on a third two men were expertly cleaning their catch. I took a deep breath to sample the memorable mixture of salt air and fish. It was a moment I did not want to forget. A few minutes later as I passed some shops, hot bakery smells encouraged me to go inside to watch a variety of unfamiliar but scrumptious looking bakery products popping out of the oven. Four or five of them found their way into a carry-back-to- the-hotel bag to share with my wife. I told her about my exhilarating walk as we ate my morning catch. I can't remember what they were called (certainly not Danish) but they were still warm, aromatic, Norwegian baked goods. The aromas of that bakery, the harbor smells, and that walk gave me a vivid unforgettable memory of Bergen.

Finding a pile of burning leaves on a fall morning is a special though infrequent treat on my walks for, thanks to today's concerns for pollution and fire, not many people burn leaves today in the gutters as they did when I was a boy. Still, occasionally when I'm away from home I pass by burning leaves and suddenly I'm a kid again in Bronxville, New York. Once again I'm helping Dad and Mother rake the leaves into the gutter. Dad lets me strike a match and set fire to the leaves at one end of the pile, in the middle and then at the other end. Mother is standing by with a hose. Smoke rises as the dry leaves crackle. It's a good smell. It says fall. It says clean-up time. Still, a killjoy friend of mine says she doesn't share my enthusiasm for the memory of burning leaves. Burning leaves to her meant it was fall and she had to go back to school. Dry leaves also have a distinctive smell that reminds me its fall and Halloween is at hand. I always thought leaves smelled best after kicking some neighbor's carefully raked pile and watching them explode into the air. It's wonderful how a swift kick into a pile of leaves can take 60 years off my life!

Not all smells are positive and one unsavory smell I encountered brought back a special childhood memory. Randy and I were spending two nights with friends in Carmona, Spain about 20 miles east of Sevilla. Spanish paradors (and Portugese posadas) are rebuilt or renovated small castles turned into hotels. The new part of our parador, the Aleazar del Rey Don Pedro, matched the reddish stone of what had been castle ruins. It looked like a kind of Don Quixote 16th century castle. It was perched on the top of a hill inside the walled city and provided a 360 degree view for dozens of miles in all directions. The sun had just risen behind a hill 30 to 40 miles away as I started my walk down the hill into the village.

Most of the buildings on the narrow streets were white or pale blue. Shutters and doors at street's edge were all closed restricting passers-by from seeing what likely were some beautiful interior courtyards and homes. Second floor window boxes displayed a variety of pretty flowers.

At 7:30 men already were sipping coffee at hole-in-the-wall cafes. I turned into an open air vegetable and meat market courtyard to watch men and women transferring produce from small trucks to vegetable stands, then started back up the hill just as a garbage truck unsuccessfully tried to make a turn. It was unable to move forward or backward blocking a narrow street and leaving me no room to pass. Not wanting to walk back down the hill to find a longer uphill route, I decided to be patient to see what would happen. A mongrel dog began barking as a horse drawn cart came up behind me. Its owner quickly got verbally impatient with the impassable situation. Then as the garbage truck started to move, its garbage spilled all over the road. A voluble exchange of unintelligible name calling erupted as the smell of rotting garbage suddenly propelled me back 55 years.

I was 6 years old and staying with my family at the old, white clapboard Pine Grove Hotel across the street from my grandfather's house in the small village of Ephraim, Wisconsin. Aunty Olsen was the hotel cook and wife of the owner. I loved her because she made REALLY GOOD applesauce. From time to time she'd even let me ring the big brass luncheon bell on the front lawn. One morning after breakfast she asked me to help her take the garbage out to feed to the pigs. It was my first encounter with pigs. They grunted at me and chomped at the garbage as I proudly emptied it into a trough. I had never before so vividly recalled that episode until suddenly it all came back to me 55 years later . . . thanks to the smell of that garbage spillage in far-away Carmona, Spain at 7:30 in the morning.

Car and truck fumes are high on my list of unattractive smells and an excellent reason to stay off main roads in suburbia and cities. Still, even unpleasant acrid fumes can spark memories. The smell of sewer gas recalls H_2S in the school chem lab. Gasoline fumes invariably remind me of my grandfather pouring gas into his outboard motor boat in Ephraim. Once the smell of gasoline on a walk was strong enough to remind me of the ether anesthetic given to me at age 13 when my appendix was removed.

While inhaling the wondrous, clean smell of salt air during shipboard walks I've also been interrupted on the downwind lap by the penetrating, unhealthy and disagreeable smell of diesel fumes spewing out of the ship's smokestack.

Contrarily, another on-deck shipboard smell is the appetite-appealing aromas rising up through galley vents. Bacon, eggs and fresh coffee smells become stimulating breakfast invitations. I like those smells better!

In 1986 aboard an 80 passenger overnight ship on the Hawksbury River near Sydney, Australia, as I rounded the foredeck during a 6:30 am walk, I grabbed hold of a sticky railing. I turned astern to find two crewmen brushing varnish on the railings. Not unexpectedly a few feet downwind then came the familiar smell of varnish that caused my mind to once again race back when I was eight with Grandpa in Ephraim as he varnished his small speedboat. The serenity and beauty of the river as the sun came up was magnificent but my encounter with the varnish smell on that walk propelled me back 60 years reminding me of many times Grandpa guided me into handyman care that lasted all my life.

Thanks to the difference in time zones and jet lag, I was up very early our first day in Hong Kong. Venturing away from the security of the western-style world famous Mandarin Hotel and the business part of Hong Kong, I wandered into the back streets and spotted a truckload of quacking white ducks arriving at the Central Market. Through a street level window, I looked into the basement below where men were slaughtering chickens and ducks, cleaning fish, and chopping up vegetables. The air was permeated with predominately fishy and mostly unpleasant smells. It was now 5:30 am and I moved on.

Further up a steep, narrow back street Chinese men and women in drab dress were setting up their food, fish and flower stalls. The view up and down the hill was a pageant of carts and colorfully decorated banners hanging from second floors. My much rehearsed "knee how" (phonetic Chinese for how-do-you-do) received broad smiles and nodding heads of approval. I leaned over to smell some flowers, inhaled the smell of fish, and was entranced by the atmosphere of this Chinese market.

Several blocks from the food stalls I encountered another familiar smell while passing a Buddhist temple. When I was about 6 my grandmother had brought me some incense from the Far East. I've always had some on hand ever since. When it burns the aroma always provides me a fantasy trip to the mysterious Orient. Now, here it was, here I was. I backed up a few feet to look into the temple as several locals walked in. Not sure it was proper to enter, I stared into a dark room to focus on flickering candles and burning incense. Behind a wide altar was an ornate screen of gold. I respectfully withdrew and retraced my steps to the hotel to share my morning adventures with Clif, our American Chinese-born guide.

And so it was later that day Clif took all 27 of us on tour back to the Temple for an inside close-up inspection of a seven foot high golden Buddha. Adjacent to it were many smaller Buddhas and to either side of the altar were scores of glowing candles and incense pots. We stood quietly as men shuffled past to light candles and pray.

My early morning discovery had resulted in a shared experience for all of us. Hoping for concurrence I announced to my wife "See what's out here by walking early?" She mumbled something about her comfy bed.

After several days in Hong Kong we took the ferry across to Kowloon and a train to Gwangchou, China, formerly known as Canton. Each car had a TV set with huge speakers at either end. We never saw any video during our 5-hour trip, but were blasted the entire time with loud rock and roll music. What, I thought, had we westerners introduced to the Chinese culture? I arrived at the White Swan Hotel with a headache.

We were to leave the next morning at 6 am, so I got up at 4:45 to walk. Not a soul was in sight when I walked through the unfurnished, unheated lobby and out the door into a cold and very black morning. Instead of fresh air, I inhaled what smelled like stale cigar smoke. It permeated every breath much like the air in 1944 in Havana, Cuba where I spent three days during B-17 over-water navigational training. It was a musty, unclean smell. A dense fog limited my vision to 30 feet. The few street lights, spaced several hundred feet apart, glowed through the light fog. It was absolutely quiet. All in all, the stage was set for an eerie walk and I wondered if I should be walking alone. Would I find my way back if I ventured too far? I began counting each street light. Inside a phone booth size shack a shadowy figure of an impoverished man squatted at curbside over a little fire he had kindled in a bucket.

The ominous silence was first broken by a dog barking off to my left, then the cackle of a chicken. Seeking the source of the sounds, I found the animals on the deck of one of many small sampan boats tied up at dock. A young boy came up from below with food in his hand to sit on the back deck where several bicycles were stacked. Cloaked in the fog, the scene was like a Hollywood set designed for a Sydney Greenstreet and Peter Lorre mystery.

It was now 5:30 am as, counting the street lamps to find my way back to my hotel, I again passed the man still hunched over his little fire. Daylight began breaking up the fog and the strange musty smell disappeared as I stepped inside the cold hotel lobby.

One seldom encounters an unfriendly farmer. Farmers don't seem to mind a bit of trespassing unless they are in the middle of a critical chore. One crisp October morning at a cross-roads farm near our overnight hotel in Burnhouse, England, I saw a 15-year-old lad finishing milking a cow. We said hello to each other, then talked about his Dad's farm, his chores, his schooling. The tousled-headed blond youngster struck me as obviously strong, optimistic, and a proud and enthusiastic young farmer.

There was a rich smell of cow manure as he started up the tractor to haul the spreader into the field. A familiar smell of gas fumes spewed forth as we waved good-bye to each other. I walked through an adjoining field, recalling my summers working on a farm. The clean, rich intoxicating smell of new mown hay persuaded me that farm smells would also forever be part of the cornucopia of memories this young farm lad was storing away.

I wish I knew more about flowers. How satisfying for the horticulturist who is able to match botanical names with the fragrances of flowers. I am forever confused. Orchids should smell; but they don't. Dogwood trees and azalea bushes should smell. So should buttercups, but they don't either. I can recognize the smell and know the name of Jasmine in Hawaii and California, and the spring smell of honeysuckle in New Jersey, and roses of course, but that's about it.

Meandering across my home Springdale Golf Course, Nugget and I stooped over to examine a vase-shaped violet flower I had watched spiral down from a tall tree. Except for its exotic look and sweet aromatic smell of the flower, it should have been an oak tree. I brought the flower home for Randy to consult her arboreal guidebook. She determined it was from a catalpa tree.

Invariably and unexpectedly each spring I encounter a similar haunting smell. When the scent catches my attention, it takes me right back to 1943, right back to HER.

As an air cadet in 1943, the Air Corps had sent me to Michigan State University in Lansing, Michigan after four weeks of basic training in Atlantic City. In this middle year of the war only a handful of male students remained on the sprawling campus with 2,000 co-eds. Excepting for weekends, they were off limits to us all, but I found a way to beat the restrictions.

Knowing there was a job available with special privileges, and knowing also how to type extremely fast, I talked my way into being Cadet Sergeant, a part-time administrative job. This freed me each night after dinner (while my buddies were restricted to their dormitories) to take the daily mail to the guys in the infirmary.

Nancy Rucker was a most attractive co-ed who just happened to live in a dorm right by the infirmary. And I just happened, night after night, to return late to my dorm, sir, because of this delay or that delay, sir. No sir, of course it will not happen again, sir. It was spring and each night a sweet, flower fragrance followed me along the walk to her dorm. Even in the daylight, I could not locate it's source. Still, to this day when I smell that smell, for a moment I am wonderfully overwhelmed with memories of my two month infatuation with that beautiful co-ed.

One spring afternoon in 1988 friends Jack and Nancy Worthington joined me and Randy in a walk through the nearby Institute of Advanced Study woods. Suddenly, I caught that same haunting 1943 Michigan State smell. Neither Jack nor I could find a thing with a bloom. Further on, we encountered it again. We even got down on our hands and knees, sniffed the grass, and weeds—looked at and sniffed at everything in sight. Our wives looked on incredulously. Strangely, we simply couldn't locate the source. Even so, each spring during my morning walks that memorable aroma returns and takes me back to a romantic 1943.

Flowers look more beautiful and smell best early in the day. It's an exquisite time to stop, stoop over, and luxuriate in the aromatic flower glories of the morning. Wherever my morning walks have taken me roses seem to be everywhere in gardens, in parks, along sidewalks and in the front yards of private residences. While the English take particular pride and care of their gardens and usually have a wide variety of flowers to smell, my luck once took me to Queenstown, New Zealand during their Annual Flower Festival. Dozens of front lawns were resplendent with beautiful flowers. Each had been carefully manicured in hopes of winning the Best Garden Award. Any one of the gardens would have been competition to Mother England's best. My walk that morning was a picture of color combined with a feast of aromatic sensations especially with the smell of roses and ever more roses. I dallied here and there as the rising sun sparkled on an early morning dew while savoring one of my most delicate, sweetest, fulfilling walks ever.

There is something distinctive, something spiritual about the smell of a pine tree. Who cannot recall the wonderment, the magic as a child staring with anticipation in front of a live evergreen tree on Christmas Eve as the whole family dresses the tree with ornaments and tinsel? Someone gets the special privilege of turning on the lights. A few presents are already under the tree "So Santa will know where to put the rest." All the while there is a strong aroma of the evergreen tree. Little wonder that encountering that smell any place at any time of the year suggests peace, family love, and the Christmas season spirit. My evergreen memories were further enhanced by the forest of pines and aromatic balsams around our tent when I was an 11-year-old camper in Maine. And so my early morning feet go out of their way to seek out the memorable smell of evergreens.

And Sounds Too . . .

In October on my 2974th consecutive day I was walking on Edgerstoune Road with Echo on leash. A strong smell of pine needles caught my attention. I stopped to breathe in the essence and write a note reminding myself about something. A few yards beyond, the quiet was broken by the sound of a babbling brook. For fun, I wondered how many other sounds

I could hear. First a bird chirped across the street. I heard a car coming a block away, heard the noise increase and fade as it passed. Caw caw . . . a nearby crow sounded off. A school bus clattered by followed by the smooth sound of a Chrysler New Yorker. Then a vintage 1975 car chugged by followed by gentle whooses in both directions of other cars as parents delivered children to the nearby Hun School.

I headed down the street to cross over the well traveled Route 206. A huge transport truck hissed in response to its hydraulic brakes taking hold. A cement truck lumbered by rattling its bulbous concrete mixer. The stoplight brought all cars to a temporary quiet halt permitting me to hear an overhead plane. A moment later came the distant sound of an ambulance with its whoop-whooping siren. I crossed 206 trespassing once again to take a short cut home by crossing the back yard of a house adjoining the Governor's mansion. I kicked up some leaves and I stopped to hear the delicate landing of a falling leaf—then another and another. On the way home I listened to the gentle foot pads of Echo as she trotted along and concluded that listening, as well as smelling, was another great opportunity for adventures in walking.

New house smells are very special and I've enjoyed them hundreds of times on my early morning walks (See Chapter on "Houses"). While in most parts of the U.S. fir or pine is used for basic construction, the smell of oak, cherry, or mahogany woods brings to mind bookcases, doors, and tables. Each wood holds its own scent and meaning. Cedar and redwood, unlike most other woods, retain an aroma even after drying out. The smell of cedar chips packed around the base of newly planted trees and bushes is especially satisfying. On winter days, carpenters toss scrap wood into a metal barrel to kindle a warming fire. The resultant potpourri of burning wood smells has a warming, ambrosia blend of aromas particularly pungent on a cold winter's morning.

The smell of newly cut grass—particularly onion grass—suggests rejuvenation and freshness. The aroma is particularly sharp in the morning. New mown hay has an equally marvelous fragrance. For me, either one is a wholesome pick-up tonic, a morning elixir better than that first cup of coffee.

I contend I can smell snow coming. But the smell of rain ranks very high on my list not for any fragrance, but for its associations. After the rain has stopped and the sun has just returned, all is quiet and fresh. The birds have a special quality in their singing. There's a peace and serenity of the new day. And the world smells clean.

The open-minded, curious early bird walker has exquisite opportunities to savor a full spectrum of the five senses of seeing, hearing, smelling, feeling and tasting. And now I've acquired a sixth sense . . . that of looking forward to the first five.

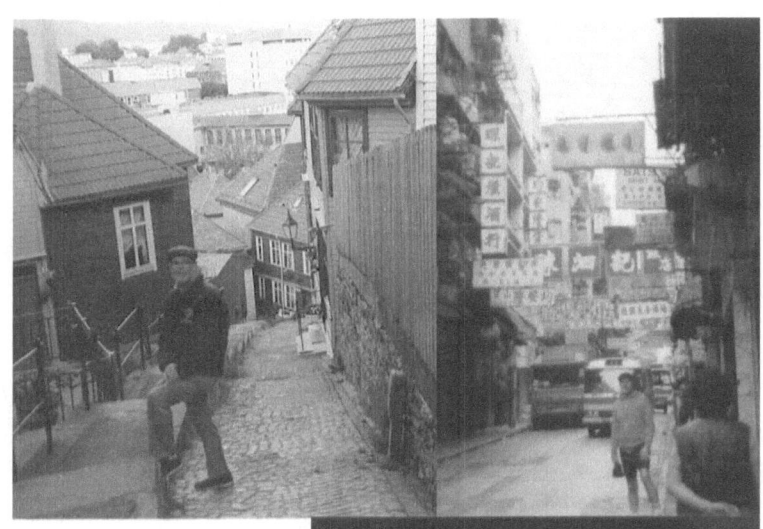

(L) Bergen, Norway
June 20, 1987

(R) Hong Kong
awakens at 6:30 a.m.
March 9, 1985

(Bottom) Atop the
Tor, Glastonbury,
England
one day before
8/8/88.

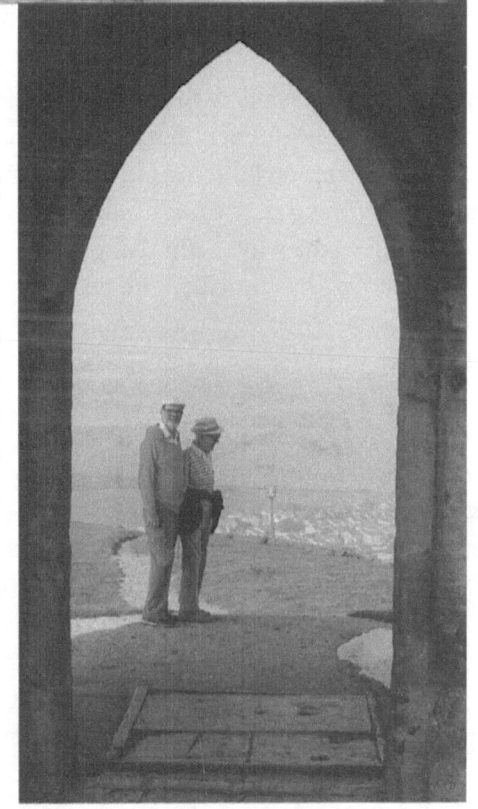

CHAPTER 5

THE GLORIES OF SUNRISES

"Getting out of bed when it's still dark might be a hard sell. Suffice to say that watching the dawn break over the ocean is a tranquil, beautiful experience. The sand on the beach is cool on your feet . . . the birds soar and dip around you and the loudest sound is the low roar of the waves."
—Bill Kent, *Shore Bets*, "Applause," August 1988

While I generally wake with the sun, not infrequently I rise specifically to see a sunrise. A 50 acre field in front of the Institute For Advanced Study administration building provides a landscape to guarantee beautiful sunrises year-round be it a hot summer sun rising from the southeast over the building or the winter sun rising to the northeast over huge trees.

This setting has provided me many breathtaking sunrises. They are never the same. Following a snowfall, the whiteness of the field intensifies as the rising sun splashes across it. The reflective glare of the sun bouncing off a sleet and ice covered field can be almost blinding in its brilliance. In the spring and fall the sun often reflects off dew covered grass.

A particularly memorable sunrise occurred one day early in November. The sky was a clear deep blue. The Institute field was delicately frosted from one end to the other. As the sun peeked through the denuded trees 500 yards away, the field glittered from one end to the other. Beyond and up 35,000 feet in the air were vapor trails of an airplane heading west from New York. It was breathtaking.

Nearby is the Princeton Battlefield Park which is a few hundred yards from our house. From the western portion of the park looking east, one can see the spire of the Institute. In between is the huge field where on a snowy January 3, 1777 the Americans won their first victory over the British. That win inspired a discouraged army to continue the revolution.

In the middle of the field is the famous Mercer Oak, a 250 year old tree under which General Mercer was placed after being mortally wounded during that historical battle. I was present with 20,000 others on January 3, 1977 exactly 200 years later when 1500 men from 19 states dressed in Revolutionary War American and British uniforms dramatically recreated that famous battle step-by-step. The ground was snow covered and cold with similar conditions as during the first battle. Since then I have risen more than once following a snowfall to watch the sun rise over the battle ground. It's inspiring to meditate at the common grave of 35 British, Hessians and Americans who died there and to contemplate how this win was the moving spirit for a bedraggled American army to persist in the fight for independence.

Echo preceded me through the shadowed courtyard of the Princeton Graduate College and out to the Springdale Golf course where a glowing reddish-orange sun was inching above the horizon. A hundred yards ahead and downhill was the pond that on a given summer's day is a frequent receptacle for errant golf balls driven from the 10th or 18th tees. Steam was rising from the pond on this 25 degree January day. In the midst of the vapor were perhaps sixty geese uniformly united as the gaggle headed in the direction of the rising sun. Just beyond the pond was the Williamsburgish old Princeton Inn, now the university co-ed Forbes dormitory. Rising smoke from one of its chimneys was silhouetted against the clear cold-blue sky. Far beyond the roof line I could see billows of steam rising straight up into the air. It had to be from the University power plant a half mile away.

The frost on the fairway in front of the pond sparkled with sunlight. As Echo neared the water, the geese, as if choreographed, slowly turned away, closing their ranks, and turning their heads slightly to keep a wary eye on us as they headed towards the far side. Stopping to take notes of the esoteric scene I heard chirping of birds in the woods beyond. Directly ahead I heard the sound of Princeton's "Dinky" train rattling down the tracks en route to the main line railroad four miles away. As its horn echoed throughout the country side I knew it was at the Faculty Road crossing. To my left a quarter of a mile away I could hear the constant whoosh of cars going in and out of Princeton on Mercer Road. A crow added a caw-caw. Approaching the Forbes College back lawn I turned back to look west to see sunlight bouncing off the golf clubhouse window. The geese, no longer concerned by our intrusion, broke ranks and quietly started paddling this way and that. I turned away, took a glance at the underbrush to see if by chance there was a lost golf ball, and continued my walk.

Mohonk Mountain House near New Paltz, New York is located on top of a 1000 foot high hill along side a picturesque pond. There are many trails throughout the 1500 acres of this old-fashioned 125-year-old hotel compound founded by and still run by the Smiley family. Some of the trails circle the lake which is overshadowed by stone cliffs and huge rocks. Atop a hill 500 feet higher than the hotel is a 105-year-old stone tower. Part of the Mohonk experience is to climb up the trail to the tower by one of the many paths to absorb a spectacular 360-degree view of the Hudson Valley.

Ida was a German masseuse who did a mean job of rubbing out sore muscles. But to some Ida was the leader who daily guided a few early risers up the hill to the top of the tower to see the sun rise. She never missed a single morning. In winter she started the half hour walk at 5:45 am. In summer it was at 4:30. Usually 4 to 10 people turned up for a cup of coffee at her brief pre-walk instructions during which she cautioned everyone to be quiet on the trail so as not to disturb her deer, rabbits and chipmunks.

This particular morning was June 22, 1986. My 93-year-old mother was hosting 65 members of her family for the weekend at Mohonk. My niece Rosemary, nephew Tad and brother-in-law Bud joined me and 4 others at 4:30 am in the lobby. Ida handed each of us towels. "For what? I asked. "For da skinny dipping when ve cum down," she responded. The early walk began to look interesting!

Instead of heading directly up hill, Ida first took us downhill. Her flashlight created eerie shadows as she led us past and under huge rocks. 10 minutes later she started up a trail as dawn's early light appeared. Suddenly she stopped, turned around, and signaled for quiet. She pointed through the woods at a rabbit staring at us. From thirty feet away she talked quietly to the rabbit, tossed it a few crumbs. The rabbit hopped forward within a few feet of her to pick up the food. It seemed to know Ida. Then, avoiding the man-made path, Ida started climbing up some rocks, squeezing herself through a rock crevice. We squeezily followed. She seemed to enjoy creating a morning obstacle course for us.

The quiet signal again appeared. There, 50 feet away, were two deer. They raised their heads, cocked their ears attentively. "Cum, cum" said Ida. She tossed out some bread from her knapsack. "Cum, cum" she repeated. The deer moved closer.

One deer cautiously took the bread out of her hand. While many of us curse the deer in Princeton for foraging and causing car accidents, the relationship between Ida and the wild deer was extraordinary to watch.

As Ida moved up the trail, the deer followed keeping about 30 feet away. She knew they were looking for bread and tossed them more. The deer disappeared and a chipmunk came up to Ida. Moments later two rabbits appeared. Seemingly all the creatures in the woods counted on Ida's daily walks and, thanks to her gentleness and food offerings, they had no fear of her nor her daily guests.

A few moments later, we arrived at the base of the tower and climbed the 100 steps to the top. A low bank of clouds on the horizon had so far prevented a sunrise. "There!" she cried as the first ray of the sun peeked over the cloud curtain. Out came cameras. The sun moved up an inch, then another and another. Cameras clicked. Within two minutes the sun was freed of its cloud bonds and was spreading its light all over the countryside. Below, the hotel was still in the dark. Far beyond, towards the Hudson River, the valley was filled with low morning fog. It was a majestic sight.

Having enjoyed other hilltop sunrises with Ida, I knew what was coming next. Out of her knapsack came medicine size paper cups followed by a bottle of her "schnapps," her concoction of vodka and apple juice. She poured a small dosage for each of us. "Sip slowly" she cautioned. It was tart but a choice reward for our early rising and hike up the mountain.

We followed her down a different route to the other side of the lake, the location of a beach and dock. "Da men to da dock, da women to da beach" she directed. Slightly out of sight of each other, the men and women stripped down, the women walking into the water from the beach and the men walking out to the dock with towels around their waists before going down the ladder to swim out into the lake to meet the ladies.

The cool water was refreshing, the conversation amusing. After our swim, a few minutes later we separated, dressed, re-grouped and walked back to the hotel. Greeting the new day with Ida was not yet over. Into the kitchen she took us to watch the bakery chef take fresh muffins out of the stove. "Take vun vile dey are hot" she urged. Into the kitchen dining room we went to eat our muffins, drink some juice, and enjoy fresh coffee. A communication with animals, a healthy hike, a paintable sun rise, an early morning skinny dip, and freshly baked goods and fresh coffee. It was 7 am. What a way to celebrate a new day!

Over the years I must have seen the sun come up with Ida 8 or 9 times, some in summer, some in the winter. No skinny dipping through the ice, of course, but always the schnapps and the fresh muffins and coffee and always her animal friends who left tracks in the winter snow. The last time I was there Ida had retired. No one at the hotel had yet volunteered to do what she had done each and every day. Still, I shall forever be grateful to Ida for showing me beautiful, sensitive, new ways to enjoy nature in the early morning world.

At the edge of the town of Glastonbury, England there is a hill known as the Tor. Ruins at the top stand silhouette against the sky. Anticipating a beautiful sunrise from the hills, I left the George and Pilgrim's Inn at 6:30 A.M. A bearded young man in Levi's directed me through the town to the bottom of the 500 foot hill.

The path—which was used as much by sheep as by climbers—had a steep incline. I stopped several times not only to catch my breath but to enjoy an ever widening scene of beauty. Beyond the town was a valley filled with a sea of low clouds spreading east and west for miles. Above was a clear blue sky. Distant hills appeared as islands rising in the midst of the gray-white sea of clouds. The spire of the Glastonbury Cathedral and portions of the ruins of the Abbey below peeked through the clouds in an ever more spectacular scene.

Below and to the left two dogs raced through a field past several cows. Their distant barks made me realize how high I had climbed. The ruins of the 15th century church ahead came closer. Dozens of sheep grazing within a few feet of the trail seemed impervious to my presence. Twenty-five minutes from the bottom I reached the top of Tor to inspect all that remained of St. Michael's Abbey cathedral ruins and its 75 foot tower. The sun was now well above the horizon and the clouds in the valley below so simulated a gray sea I could visualize a ship sailing through it. The quiet of the moment was intruded upon only by the distant whooshing sound of cars and twittering birds nearby.

I walked through the tower archway to the shadowed other side. Sitting with her back against the tower was a young girl reading a book. A few feet away was a sleeping bag with a mass of hair protruding. Beyond were several more sleeping bags. Each of the sleepers seemed long overdue for a haircut. "Good morning" I said to the young woman. "Isn't that a glorious sight below?" Her answer was "It's kind of like heaven above the clouds."

I asked what she and the others were doing sleeping atop the famous Tor. "We're here for 8/8/88" she said . . . "it's going to be a gathering here of people from all over England for a free day to share ideas for a better planet."

"How many do you expect?" I asked.

"We hope to have hundreds by for 8/8/88 on Monday" she responded.

I stepped again into the sunlight to notice beer cans and a few wine bottles, remnants of a party the night before. The tranquil scene was yet to be disturbed by the awakening of the young people who had picked this spot to celebrate an unusual date. I headed back down hill to the inn for breakfast eager to share my encounter with my wife and Nancy and Jack Worthington with whom we were traveling.

The next morning I persuaded Jack to join me to hike back up the path to the top of the Tor. The ruins now had more meaning for I had learned St. Michaels' Abbey was where Richard Whiting, the last Abbot of Glastonbury Cathedral, had been taken to be drawn and quartered when Henry the 8th dissolved the church in 1539. The view at the top was as lovely as the day before though the unusual sea of clouds below was gone.

The same young woman was still there and graciously agreed to take a picture of Jack and me along side the tower. This 8/7/88 morning there were many more sleepers than the previous day. The sheep were gone. After 15 minutes atop the Tor we headed back to the George and Pilgrim Inn for breakfast.

Before we left town several merchants observed that the town was being overrun with "dirty, slovenly, unkempt hippies scaring off business." I must admit those that were up and about on the Tor fit the description. For the young people, the next day 8/8/88 event to create a better planet must have been a success. The London Times on 8/9/88 reported over 500 young people had encamped atop the famous Tor. Townspeople had been less than overjoyed and likely King Arthur, whose bones had been buried in 1276 in the Glastonbury Abbey below, might not have understood either.

"The English walker knows the ground is alive; he feels the pulses of the wind, and reads the mute language of things. He is not merely a spectator of the panorama of nature, but a participant in it . . . Americans are . . . not innocent and simple-hearted enough to enjoy a walk. We have fallen from that state of grace which capacity to enjoy a walk implies."

John Burroughs in "The Exhilarations of the Road"

On another trip we checked in at the Izaak Walton Hotel in Dove Dale in an area of Derbyshire called the Peak District. Randy joined me for a walk along the roaring stream where Izaak Walton must have roamed and fished while he was writing his famous COMPLEAT ANGLER. Having already seen the stream, the next morning I decided to walk in the opposite direction, a decision that provided me one of my loveliest walks ever.

I set out not expecting the cool wind but, happily, I had brought along a jacket. The hotel sits part way up a large hill. The valley below was covered with early morning ground fog. Up through a field I went, over a stile, past some cows munching grass, and opened a gate into the next field. After 15 minutes of climbing a rather sharp incline, I turned to see such a stunning view that I had to sit down just to absorb it. Above was a crystal blue sky. Perhaps two miles away the tops of the hills being touched by the rising sun providing a dramatic shadow over the blanket of fog just below. This side of the fog a half mile away was a large field filled with sheep. Suddenly hundreds of sheep gathered into a single flock to race off to the east. Behind them a dog darted this way and that. Another dog on the other side of the sheep joined in to direct the animals towards the sheep farmer who appeared as a little speck at the far end of the field. This was my first observation of the incredible talents of sheep dogs at work. Too far way to hear any barking, the scene was like a silent movie, a pattern of beautiful greens and blues as the dogs herded hundreds of sheep in a cinematic interlude. High on that hill I sat enthralled, absorbing every delicious moment of a rare pastoral scene.

Unless it's raining or overcast, every morning anywhere can provide a distinctly different and, as my mother used to say, a "splendiferous" sunrise. I particularly look forward to sunrises away from familiar home locations. In March 1985 we went to China. Thanks to jet lag and required early starts by our tour group, I saw the night shadows lift over the city of Hong Kong, watched Chinese doing their graceful Tai Chi exercises at dawn in Guilin, and stood in fascination in a Shanghai suburb as the sun rose to watch a sea of humanity in morning traffic.

Our last two nights in China we stayed in the ultra-modern Great Wall Hotel in Beijing, an almost exact duplicate of the Hyatt Regency in Dallas. It is located a few blocks from dozens of foreign embassies. Standing tall above all other buildings, the rising sun bounced off the silvery structure causing the whole building to shimmer with light as reflective patterns changed every few seconds. Busses were already choked with Chinese bodies heading towards center city at 6:30. Hundreds of Chinese were walking or riding bicycles to work. I headed in the direction of foreign embassies some blocks away.

Each foreign embassy in Beijing had one or two Chinese soldiers standing casually by the entrance. I chanced being confronted by the soldiers at the first embassy by walking up to the gatepost to see the name of the country. I smiled and nodded, got a formal nod in return, but couldn't decipher the Arabic writing. The next very new embassy also had Arabic writing but also clearly said "Iran." Nearby the Australian embassy had bars protecting the first floor windows. Around the corner on a wide residential street a squad of Chinese soldiers was learning to march. They looked like first day recruits—disorganized and totally unsoldier-like. Their ill-fitting coats looked as if they had been issued by chance and their slow goose step was less than precise.

I cut back through another neighborhood to see several men and women performing Tai Chi on a front lawn. In unison, their slow motion and Tai Chi movements simultaneously provide meditation and muscle toning. En route back to the hotel a man cycled past with a young baby sitting in a basket on the front of the handle bars. The child was totally enclosed in a plastic covered housing. Very clever and very practical, these Chinese.

An hour had passed since my departure. The sun was now well above the Great Wall Hotel. The flow of walking and cycling Chinese commuters was ever more dense. Many turned to look at me. I was getting used to their stares. After all, I was the only one around that didn't look like them.

Photograph A Memory

Occasionally I take a camera along—just in case. One morning in London in September 1983 I was near Westminster Abbey and Parliament as the sun rose. Setting the camera on a bench heading east, I ran fifty feet to capture a self-portrait of me in the foreground and the rising sun and Big Ben behind me. In March of 1987 I got up early to see the sun rise in Alice Springs, Australia. It's a forlorn little town in the middle of nowhere where a hundred years ago it was a stop between Melbourne in the south and Darwin 3000 miles to the north. I knew the flatness of the terrain would provide me a sunrise unimpeded by any obstruction. Sure enough it popped up huge and red hot and provided a spectacular photo.

One 1984 January morning I saw a most unusual effect while watching a sunrise over the ocean on Florida's east coast. Typically there are low distant clouds over the water with a clear blue sky above. As a small bit of sun showed itself just above the horizon another sun seemed to be rising to the right of the first. A horizon-level cloud formation was splitting the sun in two. In fascination I watched two simultaneous sunrises as each section of the sun slowly rose. Happily, I had my camera to snap the unique picture. Though the clouds then closed over the dual sunrise, five minutes later the full sun rose above the clouds providing me my third sunrise of the day!

One of my most memorable sunrises was in Grenada, Spain. Following our 40th June college reunion, fourteen Princeton '44 classmates and our wives had spent six days in Estoril, Portugal. For six days we talked and talked, wined and dined, went sightseeing and renewed old friendships. Then Sandy and Grace McPherson and Randy and I took a driving tour of Spain. Our second stop was Grenada where we spent several hours wandering through the famous Alhambra, the huge 14th century palace that includes the room where Queen Isabella presumably gave money to Christopher Columbus for what turned out to be his famous 1492 voyage to find the New World.

The Alhambra sits up on top of a hill overlooking the city. Fascinated by my day's tour, the next morning I walked back up to see it again from the outside. Hurrying along in order to arrive by sun-up, I took numerous shortcuts through underbrush. My timing this day was perfect. The clear sky was already bright but the sun was still behind a snow capped mountain ten to twenty miles to the east. Above was a full moon. Suddenly into this scene the sun began peaking over the snow capped mountain. A full moon, a June day with snow on a distant mountain, the Alhambra along side me and the sun rising into a perfect, clear day. Would that my forgotten camera could have captured this extraordinary sight!

Queensland, New Zealand, is a town of 3500 people along a huge lake. After our 1987 arrival, Ray and Betty Bowers, Jack and Nancy Worthington, and Randy and I took a gondola up the 1500 foot mountain. A strong gusty wind swept my hat off as we took in a panoramic view. Beyond the town below was a peninsula which helped form a small harbor. A large old yacht was tied up at the town dock. With the distant snow-capped mountains at the end of the lake the scene was a composite picture of Lake Tahoe, Alaska and Switzerland. I began to visualize a route for my next morning's walk.

After absorbing the view for 20 minutes the women decided to return to the hotel. Our guide had told us not to walk down the 3 mile "perilous trail" suggesting it would take three hours. Seventy-seven year old Ray, seventy-four year old Jack and sixty-five year old Herb simply didn't believe it would take more than 2 hours. So down the side of the mountain we walked winding this way and that on a sometimes paved, mostly gravel road. A half hour down we saw a young couple hiking up towards us with a small boy about four years old and a girl about five. We stopped to visit and found out they were from Switzerland. They had hiked all their lives, and didn't think it was unusual for 4 and 5-year-olds to be hiking up a mountain. Happily for us they spoke excellent English during our warm encounter. When we volunteered our unused return tickets on the gondola, the youngsters excitedly accepted them and continued up the trail.

Fifteen minutes later a descending Japanese student caught up with us. Together we continued downhill, exchanged viewpoints about the U.S. and the Japanese economy, inhaled a strong pleasant smell of balsam and mountainside flowers, and stopped to inspect unfamiliar trees and bushes. Our descent had lasted only an hour and 20 minutes. How delighted we were we had not heeded the guide's advice! The setting sun across the lake reminded me the next morning it would come up behind the mountains we had just descended.

Leaving the hotel at the foot of the mountain at 7 am the next morning, I passed by the old yacht, window-shopped through the deserted village and took a horseshoe direction past a pebbly beach out to the end of the peninsula. The air was crisp, the sky was clear and bright, but the mountain we had scaled the day before across the bay had not yet permitted the sun to show itself. The calm lake mirrored the dark mountain with a startling clear image. At the end of the peninsula was a dense grove of evergreen trees, their roots reaching out into the water and their pine needles covering much of the ground. Dozens of minnows darted to and fro between the rocks. Looking east through the trees I could see our hotel and the old steamer across the bay. The gentle lapping of water provided a wonderful "lake" sound near a young boy sitting on a large rock with rod and reel in hand.

As the sun began to peek over the mountain, it cast its first glorious rays miles out onto the lake behind me. Across the bay our hotel was still in the shadow of the mountain. Suddenly the sun popped up over the top of the mountain and began erasing the shadow as it literally raced down the mountainside towards the edge of the lake.

The path of a cable car we had taken the previous afternoon was now in full sunlight as the sun bounced off the mahogany cabin of the old yacht a half mile across the bay. The stunning morning awakening was over as I returned through the village as early bird natives and tourists were now buying papers and food at the several opened stores. Curious about the old yacht, I went aboard to find a large brass commemorative sign noting historical highlights of this vintage 1905 steamer and several photos of 1910 passengers. The Queensland Historical Society was keeping the old wooden ship in excellent condition.

Ten minutes later the hotel breakfast room overlooking the bay provided a perfect spot for me to point out to my wife where I had been across the lake to experience a beautiful metamorphosis of night into day.

I was in unfamiliar territory while visiting my brother Ed in his new home in Glenview, Illinois. No sane person would have walked out at 6:15 into such dense fog. Visibility was at best three or four feet so I followed the curb. Realizing I might get lost, I started counting driveways. My challenge then became—how far afield dare I walk? If I strayed and got lost how long would the fog last? I turned left onto a path, heard the babbling of a brook and the warble of a nearby bird. I had been gone 15 minutes and began to get nervous. How many driveways was it to get back? In retracing my path, a driveway appeared. I counted number one, number two then three, four, five, six, even, eight driveways. This must be Ed's home. Still unable to see but a few feet, I turned in the driveway and walked up to—someone else's house. Was my brothers' house to the left or right? I walked back to the curb, backtracked one driveway and tried again. Eureka! My brother's front door—and the end of an adventuresome walk without ever seeing anything!

Many sunrises have provided me glorious mornings in my 6000 days of morning walks. Sunrises away from home are worth planning for, worth setting an alarm clock for an early rise. Capturing the birth of a new day in an unfamiliar or seldom visited spot is just one more of the pleasures—indeed the ecstasies—of an early morning walk. Whether it's at home or away, sunrises for me are an elixir of life, a spiritual experience, a tonic for a new day.

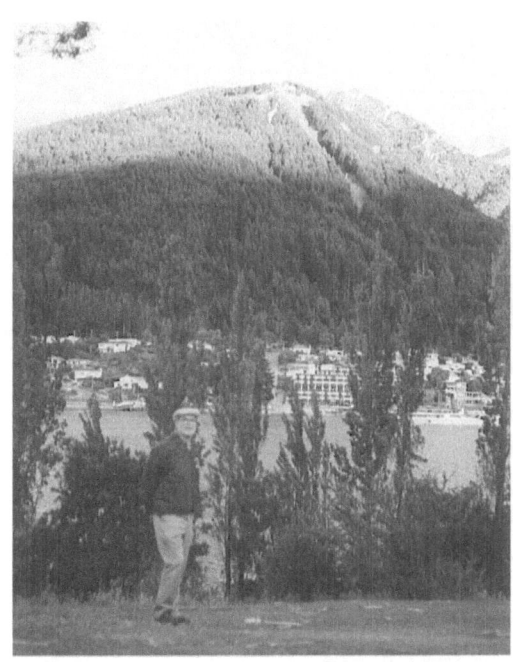

Sunrise on the
mountains
6:50 a.m.
Queenstown,
New Zealand
February 1987

Sunrise on the St. Lawrence River, August 31, 1987.

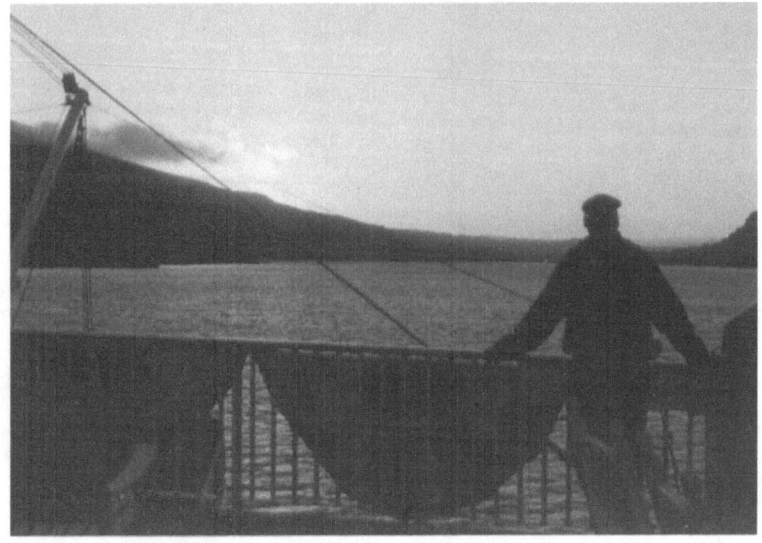

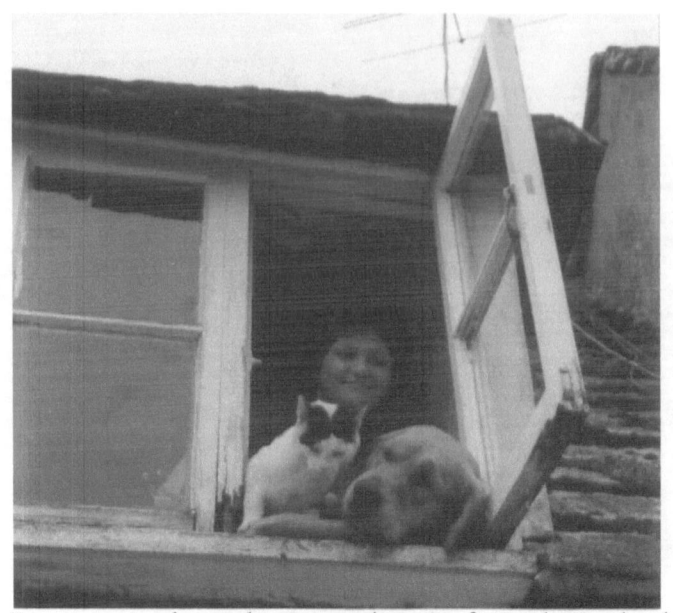

Famous animals watching passerbys, Corfe Castle, England
June 28, 1987

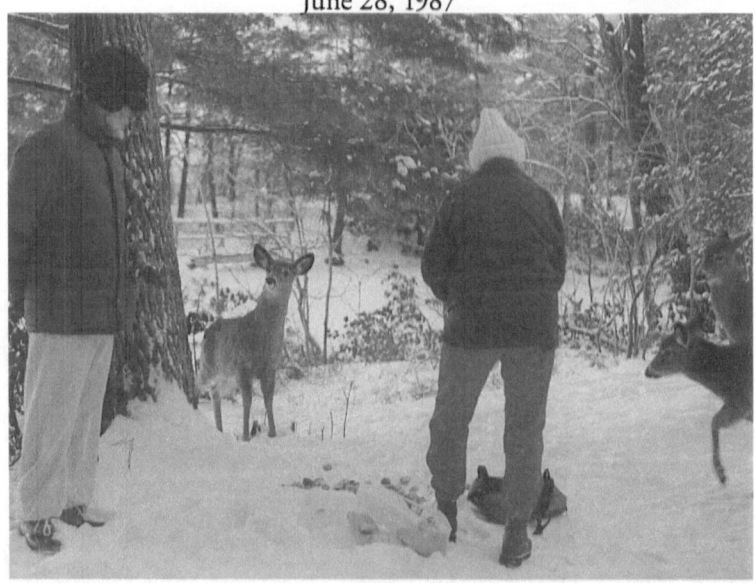

Pre-sunrise with Ida and animal friends. Mohonk Mountain House
February 6, 1988

CHAPTER 6

A DOG'S TALE

". . . you will generally fare better to take your dog than to invite a neighbor . . . . The dog enters thoroughly into the spirit of the enterprise . . . he is constantly sniffing adventure, laps at every spring, looks upon every field and wood as a new world to be explored, is ever on some fresh trail, knows something important will happen a little farther on . . ."
—John Burroughs "The Exhilirations of the Road"

My walking stories are in large part due to the companionship first of Nugget and later of Echo. It was a constant joy for Nugget to romp and chase and swim, investigate other dogs, be admired and stroked by strangers. In her last year she never left my side and my pace slowed as hers did. Hundreds of people over the years would smile at her or pass adoring compliments. That too added to the fulfillment of my early morning walks. Nugget walked with me. I did not walk Nugget. She got her exercise. I got mine. This faithful, loving and obedient dog was an exceptional companion for most of my first 2000 consecutive mornings.

As usual, Nugget poked her head in the guest bathroom hoping I was there putting on my walking shoes. She put her nose in my lap and her tail started to wag in anticipation. I gave her a hug. By the time I got to the back door my lovable Golden Retriever was bouncing and smiling at both ends—eager to have another morning adventure no matter what the weather. For six years, except for those days when I was away from home, she was a joyous companion, always by my side or running free wherever I walked throughout Princeton.

My wife and I learned to love goldens first with Clarence who was named after my father's best friend and my godfather, Clarence Francis. Our golden was so gentle and loving with our kids that we simply had to get another after he died at age 10. Jason (for the Golden Fleece) was next. He died when he tangled with a truck at age two. "Pounce" was number 3—one of a litter named after a card game. He died from a heart attack after 5 years. By now we had been overwhelmed by the tail wagging, loving Golden personality. Silence was next, Golden number 4. (Of course Silence is golden.) Silence loved everybody for 2 years. He got frightened in a storm, ran off, and was never seen again. Notwithstanding taking each of the four through obedience school, they all were loving male Goldens who were macho, boisterous, anxious-to-wander dogs. We decided to try a female next and got our Golden "Nugget." What a gentle lady! Like her predecessors, we took her through the Princeton Dog Training Club. Unlike the males, Nugget stayed at home and did not try to dig her way out of the fenced yard. She too constantly smiled at both ends. I never could give her enough love nor she in return. She was seven when I began walking before breakfast.

For some years I did not take a leash with me because Nugget immediately responded to hand or voice signals. She usually ran free, but would automatically come to my side as we approached a street crossing. When I often walked five miles on a busy road into the country to have Sunday breakfast with my mother, Nugget heeled by my left leg all the way. As soon as I got off the road, I would give her permission to take off to chase a squirrel, sniff this and that and freely explore the territory.

From the beginning of my walking streak in 1982, Nugget tagged along in every kind of weather, through the woods, along roads, by Lake Carnegie. She even went unleashed into stores where I knew she would behave. For every mile I walked she probably walked two. At age 13 she was slim and bouncy even though she had become deaf and almost blind.

Marquand Park, part of a former estate, is three minutes away. Nugget and I constantly walked through it en route to the eastern and northern parts of the town. It is also a spot where we frequently met other dogs and their owners.

That is where I met Richard Flournoy, a WWII flier and a career Pan Am pilot. He introduced me to his Springer Spaniel Doggo. "Doggo?" said I. "That sounds like a name made up by a child." "No," he responded, "that's the name for dog in Vietnamese." Thereafter, through frequent encounters, Doggo and Nugget became sniffing pals as Richard and I shared WWII stories and became friends. Several years later I heard he had been diagnosed with terminal cancer. I promptly went to visit him and, reaching for a conversational opening, I asked the whereabouts of Doggo. "I had to put him to sleep last Tuesday morning. He was very special and it really broke me up" he responded emotionally. "That same afternoon I went to the doctor with a pain in my back and was diagnosed with terminal cancer. He gave me 6 months." While Nugget would likely not miss Doggo, sadly Richard was never again to meet us on a morning walk.

The Geddes up the street got a 3 month old Golden puppy. Fanny was irresistible! Soft as a powder puff, uninhibited with wiggles and with face licking love, she was man's best friend personified. I watched her grow up as we met several times a month in Marquand Park. I'd hug Fanny each time we met and Nugget would then romp and bounce with her. Unfortunately, Fanny died of cancer at age 2. The Geddes soon filled their Golden void with another. This time they called her "Toast" to reflect the color of her coat. For the next 6 months we'd regularly meet Evelyn Geddes and Toast in the park—a romp for Nugget, a Golden hug for me. After not seeing them for weeks, I saw Evelyn at curbside getting her mail. Only then did I find out that Toast too had succumbed to cancer. It was two years before they could face up to another Golden, uniquely named Taxi.

Chris, a 5 month old Golden, Mandy, a 2 month old Shepherd, and a three-legged mutt were among many others Nugget met in the park. Having adjusted to the loss of one leg, the three-legged dog chased around as fast as the others. One morning Nugget met Ginger, a magnificent Golden—large head, strong body, obviously well trained whose owner was Sam Lenox, a New Jersey Superior Court Judge. In the years that followed Nugget, and later our next dog Echo, chased sticks with Ginger as Sam and I became good friends. One day as I petted Ginger my hand went over a large lump on her side. I looked up at Sam for a reaction. "I'm afraid she may have cancer. I just can't bear the thought of putting her down" he said. He choked up and was almost in tears. I did not see him for several weeks when to my surprise and delight there he was again at 7:15 am with Ginger. "False alarm" he cried happily. "She's okay!"

One morning as I was walking up Springdale Road my urologist Jim Varney came out his front door to get his paper and fetch his Golden. Liberty was an absolute match of a younger Nugget. They sized each other up as Jim and I visited. I noticed that Liberty stayed in an unfenced front yard. Jim explained the radio-controlled device under Liberty's collar that gave him a small electric jolt if he passed over the buried electrified "wire" fence. After a jolt or two the dog becomes conditioned to stay inside the boundaries. Like that electric fence, visiting a urologist's office can also provide a jolt. Finding out that day that Jim was a Golden Retriever lover renewed my confidence in him. Now, I knew why he had always been so gentle with me.

Once or twice a week I criss-crossed the local golf course. Invariably I'd meet Alan Poole, a Wall Street broker, and his dachshund Jones usually on the 18th fairway in front of Forbes College (formerly the Princeton Inn). Jones was a devoted and well behaved dog whose long hot-dog shaped tummy just missed hitting the ground as he trotted along. Nugget and Jones became fast friends and pleasantly tolerated each other when they met.

Alan, who at age 63 had been a small round-stomached man, decided to shape up by running. Within a relatively short period of time his paunch disappeared and he was running in ten mile races, then in marathons in New York and Boston and in Berlin, Germany. He even regularly competed at age 76 after months of recuperation from a hip operation. Short-legged Jones was no running companion for Alan but mornings on the golf course was Alan's time to walk and Jones' time to trot along with him. Sadly, Jones died suddenly at age 11 after eating some poisoned food near the course.

Two of the three blind people we see from time to time are guided by dogs. The third, a blind woman, about 30 years old, walks only with a cane but with great assurance. If we happen to meet near a road crossing, she accepts my help. The very well trained seeing-eye dog of one man hardly notices Nugget even as we pass by within two feet. I always exchange pleasantries with the man and from time to time have walked across the street with him. Neither dog seemed to notice each other. The other guide dog, apparently less well trained then the first, lunges at other dogs much to the distress of its master. During our first encounter the guide dog growled and leapt out at Nugget. The blind man, obviously concerned, shouted out "Please control your dog." Thereafter, I ordered Nugget to my side, and stayed quietly out of range.

I wish Nugget could relate all her experiences. What a joyous time she had running free, wagging her tail furiously when she met dogs or people. When she was younger she would chase rabbits and white-tailed deer and could come within inches of catching a squirrel. (Her successor Echo often did catch them.) Obedience-trained Nugget would always return on call. To keep her dry I could tell her not to dive into the pond by the Institute For Advanced Study, or the little pond at the golf course. Contrarily, while Echo had also been obedience trained, there was no way she would return on call when in pursuit of squirrels, deer, or ducks in the pond. If only Nugget could have reported the different aromas she must have encountered for my "scents" chapter in this book. I know she enjoyed that fresh muffin smell, but I wonder what she used to think of the stale beer smell in Princeton reunion tents the day after the alumni departed?

Only once did Nugget ever forget her training. It almost killed her. One day on the university campus, a garbage truck started to back up while sounding its high pitched beep, beep warning sound. It scared Nugget, she turned tail and I had to chase her a hundred yards to stop and comfort her. I didn't think about it much until some months later when another campus garbage truck stopped and started to back up. That same beep, beep, sound again scared her and she took off around a building. I yelled to no avail and chased her around the corner in time to hear her yelp and see a car hit her and dump her on the road.

Never before had she started to cross a street without my approval. It was early Sunday morning. I was a mile away from home. As I wondered if she would survive, the car that hit her backed up. A young man got out, apologized profusely that he had been unable to avoid hitting her. I picked up my 65-pound Nugget, got in his car, put her on my lap as he took me home. How grateful I was for his thoughtfulness even as he was distraught about the accident.

Shortly afterwards the veterinarian put a cast on Nugget's right leg to reset her dislocated shoulder. For two months she hobbled with the cast but continued to accompany me on my morning walks. The accident left a permanent, but barely noticeable limp that became more evident as she got older during the seven remaining years we walked together. Without her companionship I likely would not have written this book.

In the Broadway and Hollywood show "Brigadoon," Gene Kelly accidentally finds a mythical town that sleeps for 200 years and then comes alive for a day. To my wife and me, Chipping Campden in the Cotswolds in England is our Brigadoon. Each of the many times we have returned, our Brigadoon comes alive with its Cotswold stone, cobble streets, thatched roofed homes, country lanes, green, green hills, gentle streams, and the ancient stone wool market building in the middle of the main street of the village. As a base for seeing the Cotswolds, it is second to none including Lower Swell, Upper Swell, Upper Slaughter, Lower

Slaughter, and Snowshill. (How *DID* God conceive a people who could create such marvelous names?) The Cotswold countryside and villages provide an incomparable experience for walking.

One early morning in Chipping Campden I walked up to the top of a hill to get a view of the valley. A pipe-smoking man was keeping an eye on his Golden Retriever as it trotted around and through some grazing cattle. I introduced myself to John Cocks. "Sadie" he said "has been with us eight years. She's a bit on the heavy side but she's a great companion." "May I hug her?" I asked. Sadie came on call, responded to my affections and that was the beginning of several new friendships.

A rugged looking retired farmer from northern England, John was dressed with a brown woolen sweater and calf-high boots. He was all prepared to stomp through the mud and fields of early morning damp grass. As the sun rose beyond the fog filled valley we stood quietly atop Dovers Hill savoring a 360 degree view. It was a glorious, remarkably serene scene that has remained vivid in my mind ever since. As we walked down the hill he invited my wife and me for tea.

Later that day Sadie's furious tail wagging greeted us at the door of the Cock's home, one of a very old row connected flats on the main street. John and Ruth were gracious hosts for over an hour as we enjoyed English high tea—scones, jams and clotted cream and oh, such delicious calories they were.

Thanks to being brought together by a Golden Retriever, for years thereafter the Cocks and the Hoblers exchanged Christmas cards and we returned several times to visit. Their new house on the edge of town was built of the famous honey-colored native Cotswold stone. Sadie grew heavy and slow to move but continued to be affectionate. Then one day in 1991 Ruth Cocks wrote to share the sadness of Sadie's death as well as news that John had cancer. Two weeks later I wrote wishing John well while sympathetically acknowledging the passing of lovable Sadie who had brought us all together. My letter was too late. John had just died but a few weeks after diagnosis.

Another morning in Chipping Campden, I was walking along the cobblestone street and there, sitting regally in the front seat of a car, was the most magnificent large head of a Golden I'd ever seen. He was sitting up straight, complacent and unruffled, waiting for his master or mistress to return. The window was slightly open so I leaned over and said, "Hello there, Golden." The head turned slowly with a haughty, monarchy look as if to acknowledge the presence of a lowly subject. I walked quickly back to the Kings Arms, got my wife and camera and returned in time to capture the noble character of this handsome Golden.

Subsequently, back in Princeton one morning, I met a close match to that dignified Chipping Campden Golden while walking in the garden of Constitution Hill. Equally unruffled and placid, he too had a large body, a magnificent head, and a muscular looking body. Appropriately, his master called him "Bear." Excepting that the English do not approve of the darker color of American Goldens, Bear could have been a brother of that English Golden in the Cotswold whose picture in our photo album is a frequent reminder of a memorable early morning walk in our English Brigadoon.

Near Chester, England we had difficulty finding a place to spend the night. A local innkeeper referred us to a Bed and Breakfast owned by Malcolm and Pat Jones. They were remodeling their 18th century cottage and enjoyed having overnight visitors. While dinner is not normally included in B&B, they invited us for cocktails and dinner. He was a regional sales manager for Shell Oil. She was a hiker. Together they rode bicycles all over England.

The next morning I walked up the hill above their home, past several farms and through an aromatic barnyard. On the road back I met not one, but two Goldens providing me not one hug, but two Golden hugs. Upon my return we were served a hearty English breakfast of freshly baked hot rolls, eggs and bacon (English style—thick with fat), fruit, cereal, and strong coffee. A stimulating pastoral walk, two Goldens, and a spectacular English breakfast with two charming people. What a way to start a day!

Never had we been so welcome in a stranger's home nor enjoyed such hospitality as provided by Malcolm and Pat. She kissed us both goodbye like we were old friends. Two years later we went out of our way to stay with them again presuming to pay the B&B rate. Now no longer in the Bed and Breakfast business, they were delightful overnight hosts. Pat joined me the next morning and set a fast hiking pace across fields and through woods but we never did see those Goldens again. We correspond, exchange Christmas cards and have made a standing invitation to the Joneses to be our guests in the States. Besides their dream of riding bikes all over the American northeast, Pat made a condition of overnighting with us that there would be at least one morning walk with Echo around Princeton.

Nugget finally began to slow at the advanced age of 13. While other old dogs often lounge around home overweight and listless, Nugget was trim and full of pep until suddenly she became almost totally deaf. Then her eyes started to cloud. On especially warm early mornings she became listless. On cool days she would perk up.

Though quite deaf and almost sightless, she would roam free, coming right to my side as I approached a street crossing. Even as her snout had become white with age, strangers along the route would consistently look lovingly at her and call her beautiful—which indeed she was.

As she became disoriented and began bumping into trees and curbs, I had to put her on leash more frequently. She knew something was different when I took her out for only a few blocks and brought her back. She fought being pulled back into the house after a short walk for she knew I was about to take off for a longer walk. She began to bark frequently with a high pitched sound. The vet said it was senility. Her tail continued to wag as her appetite dropped, and she slept more and more. Part of my routine was to get on the floor and talk to her, hug her, brush her (she liked that), and give her aspirin by hiding it in pieces of bread. After being seen with her all over town every morning for 7 years, people began asking "Where is your dog?" I knew her time was short. She had been a devoted and constant companion in heat, cold, rain, bitter cold and snow and I wanted to continue to show my affection as she declined.

Excepting when I traveled from home, she had been at my side every single day. From the time we started our morning walks, I had walked some 13,000 miles. She must have covered at least 20,000. We had spent over 2,500 morning hours together venturing throughout Princeton.

Day by day she moved ever slower. One moment she would careen left or right, then trot as of old for a bit, then stop cold. One morning she did not come in to see me dress for my walk. I found her standing absolutely still facing into the corner of the room. She was totally disoriented. I made a decision. Pocketing several M&M's which she loved, I pushed her up into the car. My arm was around her during the ten minute drive to the vet. I talked to her all the way apologizing to her for what I was about to do.

In the vet's lobby, she ate another M&M. Her tail wagged. She looked up asking for more. I asked myself "Is this really the time? Must I do this?" A woman asked me to sign a release and I did so with tears in my eyes. Dr. Miele picked her up and put her on the operating table. He shaved a bit of hair off her left leg as I continued to stroke her. She was peaceful, stretched out on her tummy, legs forward. He inserted the needle and within a few seconds he took her head and gently eased it down to rest between her front legs. He took out his stethoscope and said "Her heart has stopped." I dissolved into tears—apologizing for my conduct. He told me it was quite normal. I gently took off her collar, gave her one last loving stroke, and walked out into the sunlight. My wife and I hugged each other when I returned home. For days we moved through the house expecting to see Nugget in her favorite places. She had been my favorite of the five Goldens, the most loving, the most gentle, a faithful walking companion. I wished I could apologize to Nugget for even thinking about having another dog.

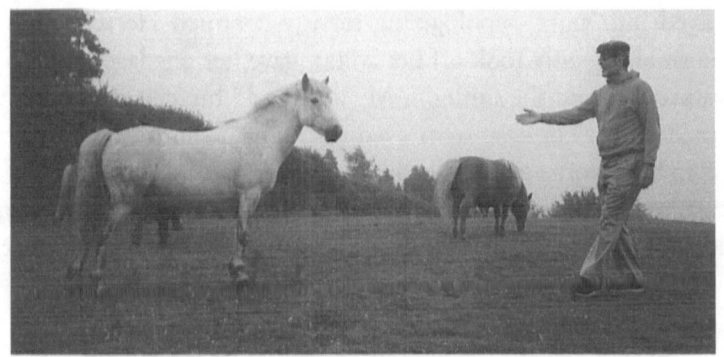

Out of the fog at Corfe Castle, England, June 28, 1987

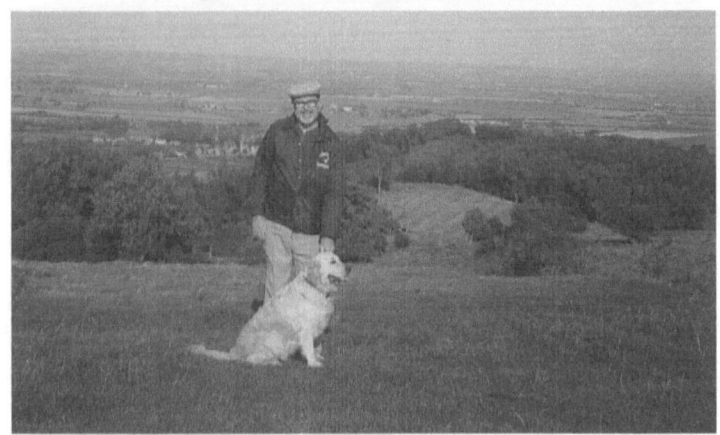

Meeting Sadie (Dover's Hill), Chipping
Campden, England, September 1982

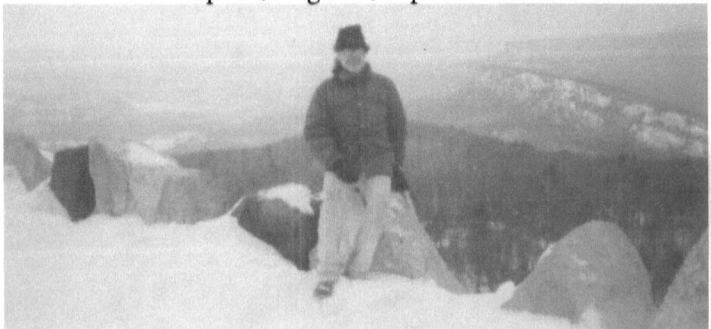

Winter sunrise over Mohonk Mountain
House, February 1986

CHAPTER 7

BRAKING AND ENTERING HOUSES

"Morning workouts are great. People who work out before breakfast will tell you there's nothing like it. 'It gets me going in the morning,' one executive reports. 'It gets my blood flowing. I think about what I have to do all day while I walk my 5 miles. I plan my strategy, create, get the cobwebs out of my mind. Then I have breakfast on the way to work and get to the office ready for anything the world has to throw at me.'"
— Othniel J. Seiden, M.D. "Walk! Get Into Shape the Easy Way"

The old house on the corner of Battle Road and Olden moved inch by inch as the huge tractor gently tugged it towards its new location near the corner. Why, I wondered, would the owners want to move it only 75 feet west from the now revealed old basement cavity? The next morning a lumbering excavating machine started digging a huge hole just east of the original house site. Was he dividing the lot, selling the old house, and building his own? The world famous sculptor of life size bronze figures was very wealthy, one of the inheritors of the Johnson and Johnson fortune. He could afford a huge home on a huge lot. What was he doing on this relatively small lot?

I've wandered through and inspected scores of homes under construction during my early morning walks but this one was something special. The third day I asked one of the early-bird workmen what was going on. "The owners are building a new house on this site, connecting it to the old house which will then become an office and working area for him." And so started a construction project that would last almost three years. After the basement and foundations were in and vertical structures put up, Nugget and I wandered through the developing house. The smell of new wood and of freshly made cement were constant reminders of the months I had spent finishing off my own home.

We stopped by every few days to check on the progress. The carpenters were always friendly and grew to love Nugget. Initially she joined me to wander through the first floor, then upstairs when the second floor was put in and later the basement. The masons were creating a charming stone fireplace in the living room. A few days later it was gone. In response to my question "What happened?" The German born carpenter with a mild accent replied, "They decided they didn't like it after all." Notwithstanding architectural advice, the owners would not infrequently change their minds once some part of the house was built—and have it done over. And that, in large part, is why it took several years to finish the home.

Four or five rooms were being created in the basement. My friendly German carpenter took me through one day and explained. "This room, with the stepped up fireplace and terrace, is for entertainment. Those concrete forms around the edges will become permanent couches." It almost looked like it was going to be a small but elegant night club. Along an adjoining hallway was a plastic panel perhaps 3x5 feet sprinkled with lights, buttons, switches, and a master control center for a stereo sound and burglary system that connected to virtually every room in the house. Another hallway led to the sauna room and men's and women's dressing rooms leading to the indoor swimming pool.

When the house was ready for the painters and floors were about to be sanded, it was obvious, with Nugget's muddy paws and swinging tail, it was time to stop trespassing. During my last inspection, skylights were in place in all the bathrooms and speakers and controls for the stereo sound were installed in each room including the bathrooms. None of the rooms in the house were huge. Indeed it was a cozy house with elegant appurtenances. While I did not know the family, some months later after they moved in I wrote "I have been in your house perhaps fifty times . . . while it was under construction. I wish you both happiness in your new home." They wrote back a gracious acknowledgment.

Constitution Hill, a former huge estate, was being developed over a three-year period with town houses. Nugget escorted me through all 50 of them as we watched progress of each from the moment of excavation to the arrival of painters. Every visit was an aromatic assimilation of freshly cut fir wood and the special smells of cherry, walnut and mahogany cuttings as internal paneling and shelves were installed. Many months later a friend moved into one and entertained Randy and me as dinner guests. The addition of furnishings and a personally conducted tour of each room provided a satisfying new perspective to the raw construction period we had explored during our early morning inspections.

Another early 20th century Princeton estate was built by the Russell family. In the thirties the main house had become the administration building of the Hun School. Now, sixty years later, the headmaster's home under construction was of special interest to me for it was to be called the Ralph S. Mason house. Ralph, a lawyer and one of Princeton's great public servants, had been on the school's board for many years. For forty years he had been a dear friend as well as a personal and corporate advisor to me. Frequently the Headmaster who was to occupy the house, would be talking to the carpenters as I passed by. It therefore was a special treat for me as the framework went up to have first hand input from him about every seen and yet-to-be-seen nook and cranny. Some months later at a small reception in his new home, the ideas and dreams he had shared with me were in place. It was almost as if I'd been part of its birth.

New homes away from home are fun to inspect. I've found traditional and modern houses under construction in Cheshire, Connecticut while visiting grandchildren, houses with a lanai in Hawaii (with gorgeous ocean views and a salty smell mixed with new house smells), stucco and colorfully painted houses in Portugal, concrete block houses in suburban Shanghai, China (I couldn't get a conversation going there), and charming cottages in England. Overlooking the ocean at Bodega Bay, California are many custom houses on all sides of golf fairways. Old friends Edd and Neil Kincaid had built a small house there. Each time Randy and I visited we saw new and unique houses being built. While on the East Coast fir is used for most basic construction, on the west coast mostly California Redwood is used. It's a pleasant and distinctly different smell than fir. The carpenters and crews were always friendly and why shouldn't they be? As they saw or nail or sip coffee, they're working in warmth, the scenery is lovely, and they have a constant view of the beach below and the Pacific beyond. For this they get paid!

On walking day 2902 we were spending a night at an inn by the water in Blakeney, in East Anglia, England. Near the end of my walk at 7:45 am I passed by a house under construction. Two carpenters listened to my story of going through new houses during my early morning walks. True to English hospitality, they stopped their work to show me around.

"Now, here's something different in English construction" said Albert. "In most of our English houses the inner walls are made of stone principally because of the scarcity of lumber. But this time we have imported fir from Sweden. It's cheaper than getting wood here in England. Note all our inside studs are made of wood. That's very unusual construction here. Wood keeps the house warmer too."

They said the inside walls of English homes are normally of stone or cinder block and with no central heating I now knew why so many English homes are cold. Of special interest to me as one who had built a lot of his own home was to note the English standard of studs 14 inches off center compared to the U.S. 16 inches. Lest the uninitiated not understand the relevance of this, the distance between studs has a domino effect on all kinds of basic construction, from doors to cinder blocks, to electrical, windows and more. In sum, like the difference between English and American electrical plugs, this would seem to inhibit international marketing of certain construction materials.

The house had a great smell not just from the fir but from what looked like large cedar beams over the fireplace and across each interior doorway. Like many English houses, the rooms were very small. "All we English need is a place for a bed and dresser" said James. He and the architect likely wouldn't make it in the States though they sure would get high marks for hospitality.

CHAPTER 8

HELLO OLD FRIEND, NEW FRIEND

"Walking is an exercise that can lift depression and cheer up anyone."
—Dr. Jane Smith, Psychiatrist as quoted in "Aerobic
Walking for Fitness & Health"

My daily walks have turned me into a well known "character" all over town. People constantly recall seeing me here or there. Some claim they can set their watch by my appearances at some intersections. (I'm really not that regular on any route.) But I do meet many old friends and acquire new ones.

Familiar Faces

After several thousand days of walking around my home town, it is rare not to see a familiar face. Some are walking, some jogging, some just townspeople doing early errands or going to work.

A half block away a New York executive left his home regularly about 6:30 to be driven into New York City. At the railroad station men and women scurry to catch the commuter train. I am not envious. I did that for 18 years and gave it up to start a hometown business. A goodbye wave at those I know gets an envious pained look in response.

When Bill Bowen was Princeton University President he used to walk to the campus from his home on Route 206. He always said hello and occasionally we stopped to visit on some Alma Mater subject. My dear friend Ralph Mason, who died in 1989, was regularly on schedule and would toot his horn as he drove to work. Lucius Wilmerding III and his wife Adela loved to ride their tandem bike all over Princeton. Winter or summer the two would briefly take a hand off the handle bar and throw me a wave and smile. Sorry, no time to stop and talk!

The person I would see most often month in and month out was early-bird Joe Sadovy delivering newspapers for the Windsor News Service. Driving down the wrong side of the road, Joe accurately tossed papers on to driveway after driveway. The heavy Sundays editions land with a big thud. We always waved and sometimes stop to talk about his ex-sister in-law who once worked in the same company as I did.

Bill Bovino once was a camper in the cabin in which I was a counselor in northern New Jersey. He helped run Bovino's grocery store and died in his early fifties. His widow Analisa drives past our house every day on the way to work and always toots her horn at me. And then there is Robert Williams, one of the boys in my club in the old Negro YMCA when I was a Princeton student. Then our six year age difference was significant. Now, suddenly, Robert is almost my age! We've remained good friends all these years and I always ask for his table at the local restaurant where he works. We good-naturedly and loudly insult each other much to the concern of nearby diners who don't know our relationship. Robert jogged almost every morning in sweat clothes and unlike most joggers, he stopped to say hello.

In the western part of town I sometimes see Mosie Gates leaving his house for work, or see Sandy Maxwell coming out to the street in his bathrobe to get his newspaper. One street over are students on the way to breakfast at the Hun School. The house of good friend and former business associate Ray Bowers provided me an opportunity to leave a note in his newspaper. When he spotted me there's was no resisting the invitation for coffee with him and his wife Betty.

Along Route 206 (which becomes Princeton's main street) Leighton Laughlin walks from where he parks his car at Princeton Seminary to his Tucker Anthony R.L. Day brokerage office on Nassau Street. An early starter, we always exchange a few words as we pass.

Visitors frequently stop to ask me for directions. One day a young woman asked how to get to the Nassau Inn. Since I was going in that general direction I invited her to join me. She was in town for the graduation of a friend from Princeton Theological Seminary and had never been to Princeton. Putting on my best Tour Guide hat, we walked through the University Campus, past the historic Nassau Presbyterian Church and, after a 20 minute walk, I left her at the front door of the Inn. Another time a name tag on a young man suggested he was a visitor to town. He introduced himself as a student at Colorado University visiting Princeton for a three day seminar.

"Do you have time for a short tour?" I asked politely. He enthusiastically accepted my invitation and followed me during a half hour talkative walk to see much of the university campus, Woodrow Wilson's two houses, Albert Einsteins' house, the Institute For Advanced Study and the Princeton Battlefield Park. The unplanned route that morning added a special dimension to my walk with the extra satisfaction of introducing a visitor to my famous home town.

It's never too late to start walking. 88-year-old Mrs. Rensselaer Lee was just barely able to walk. Yet day after day after day, in cold weather and hot, she was on Mercer Street with a nurse companion. I do not know how long nor how far she walked. I do know that this rather tall, heavy set woman slowly put one foot forward, then the other. Each step was perhaps the length of her foot. For several years a single companion supported her left arm. Later she was assisted by a second companion. But she walked—and barely walked—day after day.

After regularly seeing her at a distance for perhaps a year, I finally stopped one day to introduce myself and find out who she was.

"I see you walking along here every day. Aren't you Mrs. Renssalaer Lee?" I asked.

"Yes, I am" she replied with a big smile. "And I thoroughly enjoy my daily walk. Thank you for speaking up."

She deserved a friendly hello. More, perhaps, she deserved recognition for her determination to challenge infirmity by her daily disciplines of getting out each day to walk no matter what the conditions.

Occasionally I walk through nearby Greenhouse Drive a hundred feet away and see neighbor Geraldine Boone putting up her daily flag. She has flags of 42 different countries and, depending upon what is happening in the news, she'll fly this flag or that. It all started years ago when, while expecting an overseas visitor, she bought his home country flag to make him feel comfortable. Geraldine, now a widow, ceremoniously raises a different flag each day and uses the occasion to study the country's history. If I happen to be passing by it she briefs me on Ghana or Surinam or China or whatever country is being recognized that day.

Ed Cone, a noted composer and retired professor of music, and George Pitcher a retired Professor of Classics, live in a house next to the 18th green at Springdale Golf Club. Over the years they always walked Romulus and Remus on the golf course where we would meet. Both were very old dogs who would tolerate my younger 12 year old Nugget. It was sad to see the old dogs walk ever slower and finally become disoriented. Romulus departed at age 18 and a year later Remus died in his 17th year. For a long time while Ed and George couldn't face up to replacing their devoted companions. It was three years before they got another.

Robert Landau, who owns and operates a well known Icelandic wool store, runs every day with his Dalmatian on leash mostly in the general neighborhood of his home. In passing we always say hello but, as with most joggers who don't wish to break their rhythm, he never stops to visit. Pam Hersh lives on the opposite side of town at least a mile and a half from my house. Formerly a newspaper editor and writer for Princeton's Princeton Packet, she switched over to work in public relations for the University. That didn't change her dedication to running miles and miles all over town every day without fail. I see her running in all kinds of weather. Late forties, she is easily identifiable at a distance by her extremely erect running posture. Occasionally she will run a few steps in place in order to exchange a few words with me. Because her pace is relatively slow it's not too difficult to walk at an aerobic pace and carry on a conversation.

One morning in late October 1986 I was across town and saw a group of men and women wandering down the street carrying flags and knapsacks. They were part of a group of 700 people who had just spent the night on the University soccer field. Eight months before in Los Angeles they had started an across-the-country Peace March accompanied by dozens of supporting vehicles carrying tents, food and equipment. A bus accompanied the group to help those who turned up lame. They had walked an average of 15 to 20 miles a day while getting considerable publicity as they passed through the country. I spoke to one woman who was a 1945 graduate of Holyoke, to a man who quit his job to join the march, and to a college student. A Japanese man to whom I tried to speak didn't speak English. As I walked along with them, many petted Nugget and dubbed her "Peace Poodle." I steered my new found group of five past Einstein's house, the Governor's mansion, and then watched them disappear down the street headed east to New York.

Early morning hours are a great time to do errands. The cash machine at the bank is easily accessible at 7 am. Next door to the bank is Hinksons, a local favorite for stationery and papers. For several years Nugget automatically would guide me into the store knowing that Charlie or Bill would not only pet her but give her a whole box of Animal Crackers. That would give me time to buy a birthday card, or some pencils or a needed note pad.

On more than one occasion I'd walk from a few blocks to as much as a mile out of my way to return a discarded Super Fresh or Acme grocery cart. A grateful manager one day noted that each cart costs about 85 dollars.

Retired Professor Jerry Blum was a regular who generally walked the same route. Occasionally I'd join him for a few blocks. He was a most enjoyable walking partner and always brightened up my day with a keen sense of humor. Still, I'm not sure what he was trying to tell me when one day he told me his best walking companion was Jerry Blum—to whom he frequently talked when he was alone.

One day, just before arriving at the Squires Choice to purchase a hot banana walnut muffin, I met Tink and Joe Bolster who had been acquaintances for the better part of 40 years. They were both in sweat clothes.

A great Princetonian, he had retired from the University in charge of their highly successful Annual Giving program. They had FOURTEEN children. All arrived in about 18 years. As they grew up it was a sight to see them all packed into the family station wagon.

Even after 14 children five foot Tink weighs perhaps 95 pounds. To keep in shape, every morning five or six days a week she swims about 3500 yards at the University pool starting at 5:30 am. Afterwards she walks five miles to meet Joe who has just jogged five miles. Then, arm in arm in their exercise clothes, they have breakfast somewhere in town. Later in the day Tink works out at home for an hour on exercise equipment. They've both run in marathons and triathalons. Notwithstanding my pride of never-miss early morning walks, I stand in awe of Tink and Joe not only for their daily routines but for their togetherness.

CHAPTER 9

PAR FOR THE COURSE

"Walking is perhaps the best stress reducer known to man."
—Othniel J. Seiden, M.D. "Walk! Get Into Shape the
Easy Way"

Depending on the weather, an early morning golf course walk can be beautiful with occasional low hanging fog, steam billowing off a water hole, dampness or frost on fairways and greens, and the beauty of the rising sun over the silence of fairways. But I found early morning walks on golf courses provide an extra bonus.

A brand new ball was in the middle of the third fairway. I looked in all directions wondering if anyone would be silly enough to play golf at 6:15 in the morning. Not a soul in sight, so I lifted the Titleist and proceeded. Could there be other errant golf balls just waiting to be found?

Thereafter, walking across my home Springdale Golf course with Nugget became routine two or three times a week during the golfing season. Knowing full well where my own slices, hooks, and skyballs had frequently disappeared, it was logical to presume others had done the same. I ducked into some brambles near the 14th fairway. Thirty feet in I spotted a new Spalding. Nearby was a dirty, aged Pinnacle. I came home with 6 golf balls, washed them off and tossed them in a green plastic garbage bag for safe keeping.

Finding that first golf ball challenged me to the thrill of the hunt. During my walks I scooped up 156 of them that first spring and summer. Thus started Randy's and Herb's first Annual Lost Ball Golf Tournament. We let our backyard lawn grow for an extra week and cut nine miniature fairways 25-30 feet long (to cater to Nugget, some had dog legs, of course). Each little circular "green" had a numbered paper flag on a 10 inch high stick which became a substitute target instead of a hole. Number 9 was a water hole over a small plastic wading pool. Six of our golfing couple friends brought putters and 9 irons to play our very coarse course. Familiar Springdale golf cards were used to keep score. Then, midst cocktails and a cookout diner, most of the 156 golf balls were doled out in packages of 7 balls for the best, the worst and the in-between scores. Each guest got many of his or her favorite brand of golf balls. The golf balls of lesser quality become donations for the driving range.

I soon learned that after a hard rain storm lost golf balls in creek beds wash downstream and collect in a pile. With a ball retriever or a borrowed sand trap rake, I sometimes could find 20 to 25 balls. Once, after the frozen ground had thawed out on a warm New Year's day, a rain storm cascaded 22 balls down stream into a pile just waiting to be harvested by the Lost Ball Golf Tournament Chairman. One spring morning after torrential rains I stuffed my pockets with 44 balls and then a record 56 on another occasion. That year we had 425 golf balls to give away at our party. He who gathers the balls, of course, always keeps several dozen good ones. My 23 handicap guarantees that many find their errant way back again into woods, ponds and creeks. During my 14th year of morning walks I found over 905!. I gave over half to the golf pro for the range.

I've kept over 900 one-of-a-kind golf balls imprinted with personal or corporate names, and names of other golf clubs (likely lost by visiting duffers). A list of the more unusual of these was once published in the club's monthly newsletter that included one with a Dutchman's name imprinted on it. That prompted a call from a member who said the visiting Dutchman had lost it playing golf with him two years before!

Names on other found lost golf balls suggested some pretty good golfers had visited our club: Baltrusrol, Pine Valley, Andy Williams Open, Buick Superbowl Golf Classic, St. Andrews, La Quinta, Doral Country Club, Boca Raton Resort and Club, The Newport Cup. Business golfers left behind balls with company names like RCA (lots of RCA people live in the Princeton area), Readers Digest, Citibank, Dupont, MONY, Canada Dry, Manufacturers Hanover Westchester Classic, NYSE, and WNBC-TV. Numerous balls had company logos including a bull (Merrill Lynch's logo), Mickey Mouse, the CBS eye, NBC-TV, NFL, NL (National Lead,) the Chase Manhattan logo, and LOF (Libby Owens Ford).

Who left behind balls imprinted with a rabbit, a colorful Tiger (perhaps Princeton University), an elk, a bear (not the Nicklaus bear of which I found many), a colorful Mickey Mouse and a rear view of an Hawaiian hula dancer? Who was behind the three color butterfly and the Indian Head?

Was the "Dave Marr Pinehurst" golf ball his or a club member's? Was somebody from "Kiwanis International" visiting or was the player local? Did the person who lost "Burnetts Gin" buy drinks on the 19th hole? There are two favorite golf balls sitting at the top of all others: Who was "Too Cool Chong?" And finally as to the golf ball with the invitation–"Call me only for Sex or Golf?," which came first?

For Nugget and Echo the fairways and woods provided special adventures. Unleashed to run free, both dogs were trained NOT to run into a bunker. There were no rules about chasing Canadian geese in spring and fall which easily always escaped capture by a splash into the pond or a lumbering take-off into the air. Squirrels always escaped the older Nugget but occasionally were caught by the incredibly fast Echo. "Drop it, Echo!" I'd yell and off would scamper a startled and wiser squirrel. At other times, Nugget would leap into the water after a frog or stare anxiously at the large gold fish which occasionally appeared near the surface. Echo's loud barking at waters edge one day aroused my curiosity. There within reach of a quick attack by Echo was a huge turtle, its head just above water. The otherwise fearless Echo had never encountered such a sight. It was hard to tell if her barking was offensive or defensive. Either way it was an amusing sight. A minute later the turtle ducked under water and Echo's fascination and barking ended.

About 7 A.M. in my 7th year of golf course walking I spotted 80-year-old Art Curtiss, a retired head of RCA Labs in Princeton who was playing 9 holes. We had many common friends, had served together on the local Savings and Loan Board, so I joined him the next day with my clubs. Thereafter I became a regular by myself and in 1991 played 9 or 18 holes before breakfast 96 times and another 105 times the next year! Besides giving me a bit of extra walking exercise by rapidly pulling a golf cart, Echo gets occasional pets and smiles from the groundskeepers who are out early cutting fairways and greens and raking sand traps. True to her Golden Retriever name, she also frequently would sniff around enough to find many of my misguided shots in tall grass or the woods.

Like most golfers, I fret and grumble when shots were bad. Still, it's easier to handle frustrations and expletives at 6:30 or 7:30 am when no one else is around. Further, when early morning dampness unexpectedly slows down a putt, there's no one around to deny me a substitute shot. Only Echo knows when more than one Mulligan is used to improve the score. My pedometer usually totals from three to seven miles during a brisk one or two hour 9 or 18 hole somewhat aerobic walk. Gregory Chow, an Economics Professor at the University, is also an early morning golfer. Happily he was with me the morning my 165-yard five wood second shot landed on the green and cut a clear path across the dew-covered green into the cup for an eagle two. Echo didn't even notice.

During broadcast conventions in Las Vegas I usually stayed at the Hilton across the street from the Las Vegas County Club where an annual Men's PGA Tournament is staged. Like Bodega Bay, the narrow fairways wind past dozens of houses. No place for errant hooks and slices! After walking the course twice I was stopped and told it was private property. So much for that. However, a few blocks away is the Desert Inn. I walked it several times, once immediately after the women's LPGA tournament when the 18th hole tents and big score boards were still in place. It was fun to fantasize what must have occurred the previous day. For my golf ball collection, add one Desert Inn and one LPGA golf ball.

One of my more unusual early morning golf experiences was at South Lodge, England in Lower Beeding, near Gatwick Airport. South Lodge is an former manor home in which we stayed one night before leaving for home. The evening we arrived 20 American golfers were celebrating the end of their holiday golfing trip to England. Drinks were plentiful. Suddenly one man took his driver, stood on the grass by the back terrace and challenged his buddies to hit a golf ball between two trees 200 yards away. They were all under 10 handicappers so most of the 50 odd golf balls they hit went straight and far out into a sheep pasture. They whooped it up when half of the shots went right between the trees.

They made no effort to retrieve the balls which had landed in tall, heavy grass. The next morning along with my dear friend Gordon Fuqua (the man who got me started on my morning walks in 1982) we walked out 175 yards or so into the deep, wet grass as sheep casually moved out of our way. We didn't find 50, but we did get about 20 balls to bring back to the States to add to my Annual Lost Ball Golf Tournament inventory.

Excepting for one or two exclusive clubs—the kind with private homes, fences, and security guards—I've never had a problem walking courses. It's always easy to look like a member, or a hotel guest, or a friendly neighbor.

One night Randy and I stayed at a charming English Bed and Breakfast near the little village of Stoke Rochford. Adjoining the house was a private 18-hole golf course owned by the McCorquadale family, relatives of Princess Diana. Across the course several hundred yards away was the family's former huge stately mansion now being used as a home for the elderly. My walk took me up and down hills, past steep sand traps, near the imposing stone mansion and a stop to visit with one of the groundskeepers who seemed not at all perturbed that I was walking the course. By taking a short cut through the fairway woods I picked up three golf balls to bring home. I'd like to believe there was royal verbal abuse when they got lost.

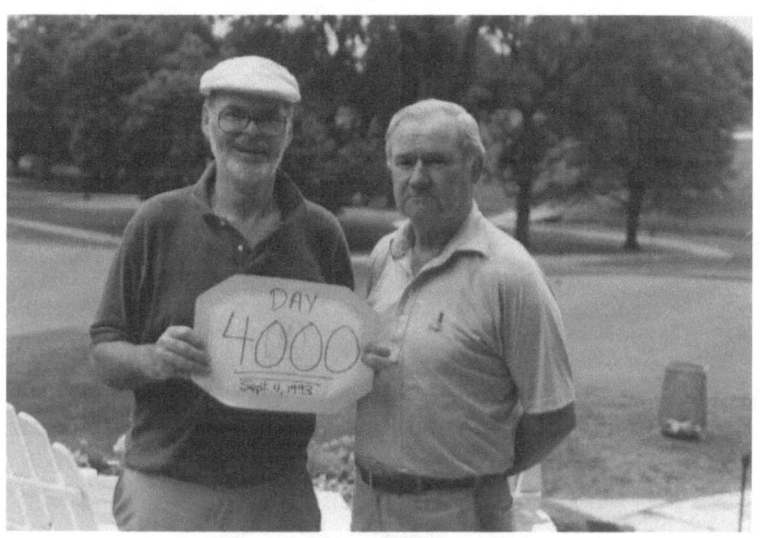

4000 consecutive mornings, September 4, 1993
with Jonas Bingeman on golf course.

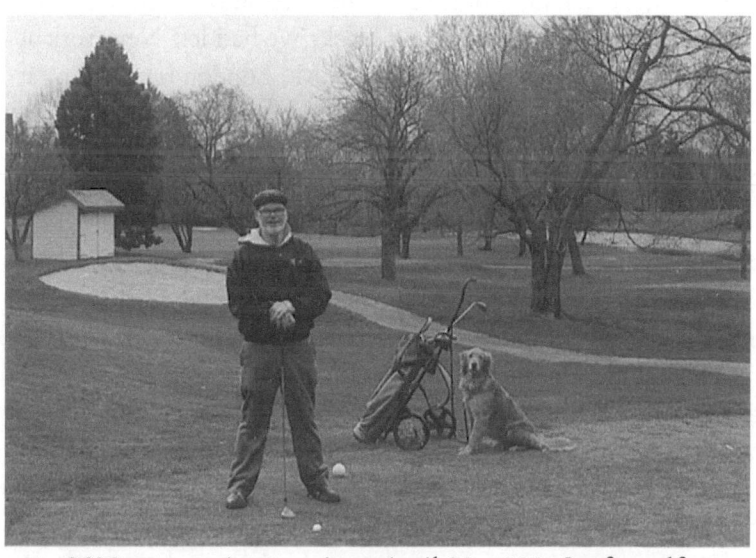

3500 consecutive mornings, April 22, 1992. Set for golf.

CHAPTER 10

TRAINS & BOATS & PLANES

". . . Walking is good for the heart, for circulation, an aid to sleep, digestion, weight control . . . makes friends . . . transforms the mind and body."
—Aaron Sussman and Ruth Goode "The Magic of Walking"

A Walk in the Sky

I leaned across Randy, who was sleeping soundly with her head tilted against the side of the plane, to lift the 747's window shade. Up ahead, just beyond the black mass of Ireland, the horizon was a glowing ribbon of orange while the sky above was still black. We had left New York at 7:00 P.M. although I realized it was really 1 A.M., London time. Now, at 5:30 am local London time, and after two fitful hours of semi-sleep, I needed to get in my minimum pre-breakfast one-mile of walking before the plane came to life again.

The routine is always the same when you fly to London. There's the waiting at the airport. Then the crowding on to the plane. There's the waiting on the tarmac and finally the takeoff. There's the waiting for drinks, the waiting for dinner, the even longer wait for the trays to be taken away. Then comes the movie, which either you've seen already and don't want to see again or was successfully avoided the first time. Finally, left alone and undisturbed by about 3:30 am London time, it's time for sleep.

Six-foot-one and one hundred and ninety-five pounds, I'm squeezed into an aisle seat. Suddenly, the domino effect starts as the person in front of me snaps his seat back into my knees. In defense, I tilt back. Within minutes almost every seat on the plane has snapped back and nearly three hundred people of all shapes and sizes are trapped, virtually locked in for the night. Tilted at sixty degrees, you have be a contortionist to extract yourself from your seat and do so only by grabbing a handful of the seat in front of you and simultaneously pull yourself up and out. This maneuver, of course, either wakes or at the least mightily annoys the person in front of you.

Try to sleep. Toss left, toss right. Push the little ineffective pillow here, push the little ineffective pillow there. Stretch out the legs. Pull them back. Cross them. Stretch them out again. Finally, with a crick in my neck and a pain in my butt, I drift less into sleep than into a kind of limbo battle fatigue. But now, with that first streak of orange light to the east, I know that it's time for my walk. I also know that the walk will revive me and take the kinks out of my accordioned body.

Timing becomes critical. Only while everyone sleeps can you walk complete unobstructed laps around the plane. If you wait until the attendants turn on the lights, you'll have to wade through the sleepy herds shuffling to the bathrooms at the back of the plane. Then the aisle-wide food and beverage carts will soon be bearing breakfast to the hungry masses—causing a complete thrombosis of the aisles. I gently extricate myself from my seat, put my shoes on and start off. I'm at Seat 35C. Having learned the dimensions of the plane, I estimate that one full lap will be about 300 feet. That means I'll need to go twenty laps to get in my one mile minimum to keep my unbroken daily streak going. This is Day 1,352 of my walking streak.

Even though everyone is sleeping I must be agile while walking through the plane. The lights are low, and many obstacles hide in the murky shadows including extended legs and dangling arms, and sometimes pillowed heads thrust innocently into the aisle exactly knee high. The bald pate of the man sleeping in Seat 45A gleams beneath his reading light. After several laps his glowing orb seems as familiar to me as a relief map of the moon. The equally gleaming—though luxuriantly unkempt—golden tresses of the young woman in 7G prompts me to fantasize. I take a dog-leg up by first class. Numerous couples are folded upon each other in makeshift shows of mutual support, and resourceful children have crafted Mom and Dad's laps into makeshift sofas. Then there is the elderly woman in 23D, whose seat is in the upright position, whose two feet are squarely on the floor, whose head rests level against the headrest (although her hat has tipped forward), and whose snores boldly ring out over the drone of the 747's big engines.

There is always a man or woman who cannot sleep and is reading a book. Usually after about the fifth lap I get a stare—sometime curious, sometimes disdainful, sometimes admiring. The stare becomes more intense as the laps mount up, until at last it transforms into a smile. Smiles also come from the flight attendants as I pass through their galleys while they prepare for breakfast. One of the great things about walking down on the ground is equally true in the air—you can stop to talk! And so, on successive laps through the galley, I strike up conversations. It's usually just chit-chat about the flight attendants' jobs or where they're from, or about my walking streak. But it's a quiet shared moment before the start of the day, a moment of easy intimacy. For a few privileged minutes airline travel becomes less impersonal.

On this flight the Captain is in one of the galleys getting a cup of coffee and shooting the breeze as I walk through. After talking a bit, we discover that he's a good friend of Lloyd Welken, the pilot of "Betsy," the B-29 I served on as navigator during the raids on Japan in 1945. (As a result, the Captain had Randy and me come up to the cockpit after we landed at Heathrow. I was awed by the advances in the electronic navigation equipment. To think that Orville and Wilbur got us up in the wild blue yonder only eighty years ago.)

I finished twenty laps—or had I lost track at eighteen or nineteen? I checked the pedometer on my belt. It registered nine-tenth's of a mile. Needing another couple of laps, I picked up my pace arriving back at Seat 35 C a few minutes later. Carefully grabbing the back of 34C, I shoe-horned myself back into my seat. Perfect timing. A moment later the lights popped on and breakfast carts started down both aisles. Seats snapped upright as my fellow passengers started coming back to life little realizing that a night walker had been watching them during the last half-hour.

I've had eight or nine flying walks before breakfast but one was most unusual. We were flying back from Australia (Day 860). I started my walk at 6 am on Tuesday and finished it the day before at 6:30 P.M. on Monday. That happened, of course, when we crossed the International Date Line.

An Elegant Walk On the Orient Express

When Randy and I had asked whether she wanted to come, my 90-year-old mother had chirped, "Sure, I'd like to go to Europe just once more. You know my first trip over was in 1910 when I was seventeen."

We began our trip by meandering for several days through East Anglia in England, staying at charming inns and then flew over to Venice. Our hotel, the Europa-Victoria Hotel is right on the Grand Canal. That first afternoon Randy and my mother walked past shops, over canals, and past hundreds of Venetians and visitors of every size and shape till we arrived at the famous St. Marks Square. Mother kept up a remarkable pace. On the way back as mother moved forward to step down several steps into a gondola the gondolier offered his hand for support. "No, thank you," she said. I don't need help." She then literally jumped into the long black boat!

Angelo poled us through one narrow canal after another. He pointed out the house where Mozart had lived and another which had been the home of Marco Polo. Venice was like everything I had ever seen in movies—dirty water, eroding stone supports under buildings, people leaning out open windows over flower boxes, arched bridges, and dozens of gondolas coming this way and that. Naturally the gondolier sang for us and we argued a bit at the end whether his fee should be 40,000 or 50,000 lire.

Two days later her ninety-year-old hands slowly reached out and firmly grasped the polished steel handles up on the side of the Orient Express. It was departure time from Venice as mother tried to pull herself up the three very steep steps onto the train. I saw she was struggling. Sixty years ago my mother had often sharply applied her hands to my fanny with disciplinary impact. Now it was my chance. I placed both my hands on her fanny, and gently *PUSHED*. One, two, three—and up she went aboard the gleaming train! She smiled back and exclaimed "Thanks, I needed that !".

We were escorted down the red-carpeted hallway to our rooms by a blue and gold uniformed crew member. Everything was sheer luxury. The staterooms were paneled in highly polished rosewood and the bathrooms were stocked with Evian water, crested glasses, thick monogrammed VSOE towels and "Orient Express" toiletries of every conceivable type. Of course, the closets had plenty of brass hangers. A fold down mahogany writing table provided a resting place for my daily diary. As we unpacked, a handsome uniformed man in his thirties stopped in to say, "I'm Christian, your steward. I'll be available all night and tomorrow any time you need me. Just call." We looked forward to being coddled.

Soon it was time for a formal dinner (at extra cost to the considerable train fee) in the opulent dining car with its exquisitely set tables covered with starched white linens. We looked at the other diners fantasizing that we were part of an Orient Express Agatha Christie mystery. Perhaps the mysterious Asian man wooing the stunning blonde was a spy? And that man over there in the corner seemingly reading the newspaper held close to his face, perhaps this was Hercule Poirot himself missing not a single detail about us all? Reality returned as the menu appeared. First there was savory pigeon eggs, then Dover Sole, while the meal was finished with espresso, assorted cheeses and thin sliced prunes. All this was accompanied by a fine wine provided for us by the resplendent sommelier complete with a pendant brass tasting cup. We took an extra coffee in the lounge car and listened to the pianist. While we knew we were passing through the magnificent Alps, nearly the entire trip occurred at night. So, our dining car windows served only as mirrors of the glories of wood and brass and crystal within.

Later when we turned in for the night the covers had already been turned back by Christian who left gold-wrapped chocolates on our pillows. The bed linen was soft, the road bed was smooth. I switched off the overhead light to listen to the lullaby of the tracks . . . clickety-clack, clickety-clack, clickety-clack, clack-clack. The sound took me back to the adventure of my first overnight train ride at age 8 with my parents from New York to Chicago when, thanks to the flip of a coin, I got the lower berth. I remember not sleeping then so I could lift the shade to see the lights of Pennsylvania and Ohio towns passing by. It was especially exciting to raise the window so that the clickety-clack sound roared even louder while letting me smell the engine coal soot as it splashed all over my Pullman bed. But that was sixty years ago and this was now, a memorable experience aboard the famous Orient Express.

Knowing we would be pulling into Paris about eight in the morning, I got up around six-thirty, had my usual glass of water (without the lemon this time) and set out for my walk with overnight childhood memories fresh in my mind. All I needed to keep my streak alive was one mile. That would have to be five or six lengths of the train? I headed towards the engine.

The door at the end of the car automatically opened to the loud sound of clickety-clack between cars, causing me to recall another memorable time that I walked through a famous train.

It was 1938. The cars between the Super Chief opened with the twist of a handle. I was 15 and going to California with a young orchestra leader and not yet widely known composer named Meredith Willson and his wife Peggy. Meredith had been hired by my father's advertising agency to lead the orchestra on the weekly Maxwell House "Good News of 1938" that succeeded the popular Maxwell House Showboat. En route from England to Hollywood he had spent the weekend at our home in Connecticut where I'd been an unwilling, unpaid hired hand that summer on my Dad's cow farm. His presence provided me a long-shot opportunity.

"Boy, I'd sure like to go to Hollywood, Dad." It seemed an unthinkable dream until Meredith responded.

"Hobe, why not let him come with me? He'll have a good time and we'd enjoy having him for a couple of weeks."

"Can I Dad? Can I?" pleaded the young piano player who himself wanted to be a composer.

Now we were on the Super Chief two days out of Chicago arriving at the Pasadena Station. For two weeks I'd wake up on the living room day bed to watch Meredith and his young arranger Carmen Dragon preparing music for the Thursday night radio show. It was a dream come true for a young movie fan to go to the NBC studios and meet Dick Powell, Mary Martin, Spencer Tracy, Robert Young, George Raft, and Ray Milland, all stars on the first two shows I watched. On the next show it was Charlie Winninger (who had played Captain Henry on Showboat), Ralph Morgan, his brother Frank Morgan (who shortly was to become the Wizard of Oz), Jack Haley (who was about to become the Tin Woodman), and George Murphy, then an actor, later a U.S. Senator with whom many years later I was to have brief business dealings.

What more could I possibly dream of except ask a presumptuous question?

"Meredith, you know all the stars. Could you get me a date with someone like Deanna Durbin, Bonita Granville, or Judy Garland who have been on your show?"

Meredith's "I'll think about it, Herbie" response didn't sound encouraging.

Two days later he announced I was to have a date the next night with Judy Garland! Meredith and Peggy took me to the famous Victor Hugo to meet Judy and her mother. We had dinner and I danced her around for the better part of three hours. It was August 28, 1938. We were both 15. (She would begin making the Wizard in one month.) And as if having such a date wasn't enough who else was at Victor Hugos that night but Eddie Cantor, Rochelle Hudson, Al Jolson and Ruby Keeler!

At the end of the evening I shared with Judy that I collected ashtrays—the cheap glass kind with the name of the hotel on it. There in the middle of the dining table was a silver plated ashtray, the kind with the small silver wooden match box holder standing up in the middle.

"I would not dare take that" I said.

"I will" she said. She tucked it under her mink wrap, said goodnight to the maitre'de and handed it to me as we said goodbye outside.

That was not quite the end of my Hollywood star gazing. The next night I met Alice Faye, Fanny Brice, Helen Westley, and Mickey Rooney. It was from those beginnings that I enjoyed a life long affectionate relationship with Meredith that included taking my family to visit him several times in Los Angeles, sitting in the third row opening night at his "Music Man" on Broadway, and having him to my home in Princeton.

I never had contact with Judy again. I doubt she would have remembered our escorted date that evening. But my silver plated ashtray from Victor Hugo has held a distinguished display spot in our home ever since.

A sudden shake of the train tossed me against the side of the car jolting me out of my Hollywood reverie back to the Orient Express. I concentrated on my balance and moved forward to the next car. Clickety-clack, clickety-clack and I was in an empty diner. Waiters were in preparation but breakfast was not yet being served. Five cars later I saw the back of the engine. There could be no further forward progress.

On my way back towards the rear of the train I passed our always-available-for 24-hours Christian who eyed me with amusement. "Good morning, Christian," I said. "I'm on my morning walk and need to walk a mile. How many cars to the rear engine?" "About six including the club car" he replied. I stopped to watch as he transformed a two bedroom stateroom back into a tidy, elegant parlor. With quick decisive moves the beds disappeared into the wall, the basin folded up, and the upper bunk transformed itself into a curved ceiling. It was accomplished with rhythm and finesse.

Just as I reached the last car the sun popped over the horizon. The countryside raced by, farm and town and farm and town. The train started to slow and the landscape became more densely urban as we approached Paris for a brief stopover.

Almost no one got off the train at the Paris station except me for I hadn't done my mile of walking yet. I had fifteen minutes to "see" Paris which I did by striding up and down the platform while catching glimpses of the skyline. I could see no Eiffel Tower, no Left Bank, no Notre Dame. But there was something distinctively Parisian about the beaux arts mansard roofs that crept into view. The conductor bellowed out "En Voirture!" That was my clue to climb back on and return to our stateroom just as Randy was rising. On this Day 325, my pedometer recorded a very unique 1.8 mile walk.

Knowing the early sunrise in England in June would help wake me, I had purposely opened the porthole curtain the night before. The sun hit my face at four-thirty in the morning. For an hour and a half thereafter the vigorous pitch and roll of the three hundred and fifteen foot long ARGONAUT alternately woke me and lulled me back to sleep. By six o'clock I decided it was time to throw on some warm clothes and venture on deck for my morning walk on Day 2008.

Under a pale sky the seas southwest of Southhampton were swept by whitecaps in the freshening breeze. One hundred and twenty-seven Princeton University alumni and spouses, including five professors, had boarded the ARGONAUT at Southhampton the previous evening for a twelve day educational voyage around the British Isles. Nary a one of them was in sight now as I headed towards the bow on my usual counter clockwise circuit around the ship. I worked to gain my balance as the ship rolled to port and then to starboard. What I had not anticipated was that walking to the bow would be always slightly uphill while heading towards the stern would be downhill. These inclines, compounded by the constant up and down pitch of the boat, would first give me a lift up and alternatively take the deck out from under me. It was fun developing a kind of hesitation walk in between steps to adjust to the pitch and roll.

The clean salty air was invigorating. I had checked the evening before to find that the main deck required eleven laps to the mile. No one else was on deck at 6:15 A.M. as I lunged and lurched about the deck gaining steadiness with each lap. By 6:45 three or four people arrived on deck including a woman still in her night-robe who was helping herself to coffee and Danish in the aft lounge. After several more laps five or six additional passengers arrived in the lounge. The first woman, still in her night robe and bedroom slippers, was now out walking slowly around the wind-protected pool, coffee cup in one hand, sweet roll in the other. As we were all "Princeton" family we exchanged morning pleasantries.

The breezy fifty-degree salt air and the rhythmic movement of the boat provided an exceptional walking experience. A door opened and a man popped out on deck. He too was a little unsure how to handle the rolling of the boat and took off ahead of me. Something about him was familiar. Was it my college classmate, Dr. Charlie Clarke, whose name I'd seen on the passenger list? With sea legs now under me, I lengthened my stride towards him. I hadn't seen Charlie in forty years. He had been only a casual college acquaintance so I was a bit hesitant about approaching him to ask "Are you Charlie Clarke?" When I caught up with him a lap later he solved the problem and said, "Hi, Herb!"

We had the deck to ourselves for several quick laps. My new-found soft-spoken old friend had a droll sense of humor and struck me as particularly thoughtful and wise. Father of five daughters, we found we had common interests in music and community service. He struck me as a reliable, old-fashioned homespun doctor. He was in good shape and kept up a good pace for a half hour. After Charlie went below deck I continued on to complete three and a half miles round and round.

When the travel group had gathered the previous evening for orientation for the first of our lectures, we'd been briefed by a tall, handsome, kilted Scot who reported we'd likely get a chance to see Elizabeth, the Queen Mother (or Queen Mum as she was known to all). She was to be at our first stop, the Isle of Tresco, the best known of the Scilly Isles, where she would dedicate a bench and a tree.

The next morning as we were having breakfast the Argonaut dropped anchor off Tresco. Shortly thereafter we all went ashore by tenders. Our tour guide took us through fabulous gardens which included some unexpected subtropical palm trees. (At fifty degrees north latitude, Tresco is bathed by the equatorial waters of the Gulf Stream). Advised we were now going to be on our own for an hour and a half, Randy and I strolled up a country lane with no particular destination in mind.

Soon we came upon a small quaint cottage, its doors thrown open to the summer air and bearing "COME IN!" welcoming signs. Inside a tall man wearing a long smock was at an easel putting the finishing touches to a vivid painting depicting a World War II destroyer plowing through rough seas. John Hamilton was obviously an accomplished painter. We learned he had spent several years on Tresco in order to create more than a hundred and seventy oil paintings of British warships doing battle in the European and Pacific theatres. He said his paintings were to be part of a book entitled *WAR AT SEA: 1939-1945*. I immediately gave him my address and a check. Many months later when it was published his magnificently illustrated book arrived with a personal note acknowledging our visit.

A half hour later as we ate our dessert on the Island Hotel terrace overlooking the water, the four-hundred foot, jet black, Royal Yacht Britannia swept into view around the far point. It dwarfed all other ships and boats in the harbor. As we started down to the two hundred foot long wharf to join with the islanders to greet the Queen Mum, a black tender headed towards shore with British sailors standing on bow and stern.

The crowd buzzed as she stepped off the tender accompanied by an entourage of five gentlemen. The several hundred natives and Princetonians instinctively formed a corridor along the wharf that spilled over on the shore where we stood. The Queen Mum bowed graciously, shook hands with the local dignitaries and then slowly made her way along the dock. She stopped occasionally to chat with other Princetonians. She walked off the wharf and suddenly was standing right in front of me. Sensing an opportunity, I spoke up.

"We are more Princetonians."

"Ah yes, how many of you are there?" the Queen Mum inquired.

"About one hundred and twenty," I replied, forgetting to say "your Majesty." I realized I was informally dressed, hardly the clothes for chatting with royalty. Still, it appeared I had her attention.

"I understand that you are sailing completely around the islands," she offered.

"Yes, we are," I said. Then, totally uninhibited, I quickly added, "I thought you might like to know that I have asked all of my friends on this trip to show me proper respect because my middle name is Windsor."

This brought a delicate royal smile from the little lady with the big hat whose royal family is known as the House of Windsor with no genealogical bloodline connection to the name. With her practiced and gracious royal nod she said, "I think that is nice." A dour escort forced a smile as the Queen Mum moved on. One tall, distinguished, mustached gentleman stayed behind for a moment to chat with me. Months later a fellow Princeton traveler, Phil Schaff, sent me a picture of this exchange. There, facing the camera, with beard and mismatched clothes and a beaming smile is Herbert Windsor Hobler. And there, with her back to the camera, is a diminutive old lady wearing an enormous hat. No need to see the face. She's instantly recognizable in my treasured photo.

The second morning was misty and rainy. I tossed on rain gear and walked with a fellow Princeton Tiger as the Argonaut slowly entered the harbor of Glengariff, Ireland. (Sadly, it rained all that day, and my first impression of Ireland was mostly deep green and gray mist.) The fourth morning we headed north out of Dublin into the strait between Ireland and England. As I walked around B Deck I wondered where we were and ducked inside to look at the maritime maps posted in the main hallway. The island of Islay was to port and the island of Jura to starboard. The two low, bosomy hills up ahead were the Paps of Jura. I couldn't help but chuckle at the thought of some poor sailor's fevered imagination that led to the name.

The timing of my walk on the fifth day was perfect. While others slept, I watched as we entered Portree Harbor on the Isle of Skye. To starboard was a startling duplication of Diamond Head in Hawaii. Shaped the same, but several miles long, it sloped from its peak at the port's entrance down to sea level at the town's edge. I ran downstairs and got my camera to capture the sight.

My most memorable walk aboard the Argonaut began on the sixth day. The sun woke me at five, I was up at 6:30, and by seven I had already walked a mile in the cool weather when Tom Eglin appeared on deck in front of me. Lengthening my stride, I soon caught with him and together we began to walk and talk.

During different years, Tom and I had been on the Princeton track team alumni. He was now a dean at the Lawrenceville School four miles west of Princeton. Although I had always admired him we had only been casual acquaintances. That was soon to change. Lap after lap that day we talked and talked about Princeton and Lawrenceville, about my walking and his running, about all the sights and experiences on our cruise, about my wife Randy and his energetic, athletic wife Edie. At every lap we passed Edie on the foredeck with several other women working through rigorous calesthenics.

The next morning was equally cool, prompting the two of us to walk vigorously as we resumed our conversation from the day before. As we passed the pilot house the captain waved for us to come in. While all passengers were invited to come in at specified hours to see how the ship operated, we got special early morning treatment. My World War II navigational experiences prompted lots of questions about the new technologies and a comparison of maritime and celestial charts. Each day

Tom and I continued to walk together. We watched the Argonaut sail into the Shetland Islands on Sunday morning, into Aberdeen the next day, and into Leith Harbor near Edinburgh a few days after that. I felt ever more privileged getting to know this quiet, slight, thoughtful, and sensitive man.

Four months later he was stricken with a brain tumor. Had I not met Tom in this special way and experienced the kinship of walking together, I would not have been among the legions of his concerned friends during his illness. The prognosis was that he had but a few months, yet Tom beat the odds after trying a new treatment at the Huntington Hospital in Pasadena, California. He lived two more years.

The 152 foot Great Rivers Explorer was small enough to pull right up to glaciers, the perfect ship to explore Alaska. Randy and I were taking a cruise with some friends heading up the Alaskan coast on a four day trip to Ketchican. Due to jet lag I had risen early and began a three-hundred foot long circuit around the deck before breakfast. It was July and even at five in the morning the sky was bright. The air was skin-tingling cool. The shoreline was barren and rocky. As had happened on the Argonaut in England, the captain invited me in to the pilot house. While he briefed me on the ship's radar, electronic gear and navigational equipment, he poured me a cup of coffee. A mile away a large steamship passed by. During this prime tourist season, the captain informed me, the big ships carry eight hundred to nine hundred passengers. By comparison, our small ship with only 80 passengers provided a special intimacy not possible on the large ships.

Our traveling companions Dudley and Polly Woodbridge arrived up on deck as we approached the tiny town of Wrangel. The harbor had twenty-seven foot tides and now, at low tide, we found ourselves looking straight up to the old planked dock. Wrangel had been a pioneer town, complete with gambling, boozing and "ladies of the evening." High up on the dock, were three such ladies (local housewives we later learned) decked out in the most sinful of 1890's fashions. Dudley and I quickly climbed up the steep ladder to put our arms around "the ladies" as our wives snapped photographs. We wanted to show the boys back home what a time we had in Wrangel!

On the third morning, the wind chill must have been twenty degrees. The sky was clear and the sea was whipped by the wind. Around and around I went, head up going downwind, and bent over from the waist bucking into the headwind. Suddenly—in the middle of nowhere—the

Explorer cut its speed and began to head to shore. Why would we stop at such a desolate spot ? There was no sign of life anywhere. Beyond, smoke was coming out the chimney of a north-woods lodge nestled among tall trees near the shore. As the ship came in closer a uniformed woman came out of the lodge, moved quickly to the dock and came aboard. Chris was a park ranger who would guide us that day through fjords and glaciers and this was Bartlett's Cove, her summer home for four months each year.

Hearing we would leave in twenty minutes, I quickly followed a path behind the lodge to explore the woods. What I saw caused me to rush back to get Randy. The two of us stole an all too brief walk through a forest, with huge fern clusters, thick moss on the northside of all the trees, fallen trees in various stages of decay, and morning sunlight filtering through the huge evergreens dispersing the wispy early morning mist. It was a pristine forest unlike any I had ever seen. If only that clean crisp air could be bottled to take home!

After the ship pulled out and breakfast was over we gathered on the fore deck to hear Chris introduce us to the area. In her mid-twenties, with bright red hair and a trim figure, Chris had a contagious enthusiasm. She pointed out the floating "bergies," little icebergs dirty with the gravel the ice had picked up over hundreds of years. The ice chunks grew larger and larger and we headed north towards the glacier. The Explorer coasted to a stop close to a small rocky island permitting us to get close views of kittiwake birds, cormorants and black and yellow puffins. The puffins flew off the rocks, dove into the water and vigorously swam away. (It was a "must" thereafter to buy a soft toy puffin to take home.) Sea otters lolled on the rocks looking up at us with quizzical expressions. Chris identified each and every species for us, including the scooters who flew on top of the water at incredibly high speeds. A passenger asked about the marbleized appearance of the rocks. "Bird droppings," she informed us with a hearty laugh. A half hour had gone by, it was freezing on deck, and more than a few of us had gone inside for warmth. But Chris got on the PA system, calling out: "Come on back to the foredeck, folks. It's so beautiful here— and you won't be back!" We eyed each other sheepishly. She was right. We might never again enjoy such an experience. Back out on deck we went to freeze, to listen and to learn.

The three-quarter's of a mile wide Margerie Glacier was now dead ahead. Under the gray overcast sky it was an eye-arresting mixture of dull white and glowing aquamarine blue, the bluish tinge coming from the encapsulated stone and gravel. A mile to the right was a dirty, gravelly glacier known as the Grand Pacific. Small icebergs known as "growlers" glided by as ever larger bergs filled the water around us. The Explorer pulled up to one section of the glacier as a long landing ramp strapped to the top deck was lowered off the bow. Extending out fifty feet, the ramp came to rest on the glacier permitting us to walk right off the ship on to a great field of ice. There is a sense of history and mystery standing on a glacier thousands of years old. Still, they constantly are being eroded as sections of ice fall away to become bergs or bergies. Chris enjoined us from taking souvenir samples of ice or stone.

The ship backed away from the glacier and began to drift slowly to a point about a quarter of a mile away. There Chris alerted us to look for huge sections of the 180 to 400 foot high glacier as they frequently break away from the main body. It's called "calving." Sure enough, in about fifteen minutes someone shouted: "Look to the right!" A giant slab of ice, seemingly in slow motion, snapped off the glacier and plunged into the water. Several seconds later the air boomed a thunderous sound of the tear and splash into the water. It was an awesome sight and sound.

"The danger of getting too close to the glacier," Chris noted, "is that calving causes huge waves to roll out. They can swamp a boat even of this size." She noted the on-going calving had caused the glacier to recede sixty-five miles in the last twenty years, nearly two feet a day. That, of course, meant the creation of sixty-five miles of new land and inlets, many adjustments for the land and sea wildlife, and constant map changes for the cartographers.

Kirkenes, Norway is as desolate a town as I have ever seen. With the Arctic Sea on one side and totally barren rocky low hills on the other, it looked, even in June, as though nothing could possibly grow anywhere. At seventy-three degrees north—three hundred miles north of the Artic Circle—it was barren.

The seven hundred mile flight on SAS from Fornebu Airport just outside of Oslo north to Kirkenes had been a high altitude preview of beautiful things to come.

Most of the flight was over Sweden. An hour out we were over snow capped mountains as the pilot first pointed out Finland to our right and a few minutes later announced "That is Russia now on our right. No photographs may be taken." What, I wondered, could a tourist camera possibly see in Russia at this altitude ?

Our Kirkenes busses took us to the aptly named Tourist Hotel on a hill overlooking the town. The 1987 summer midnight sun period had started May 29th just a few weeks earlier. We sat down to a ten o'clock dinner with sunlight pouring in the dining room window.

I tossed and turned all night (or should that be all day?). Part of the problem was sleeping under the comforter-like loose duna that constantly exposed my feet. Why couldn't the Norse have sheets and blankets that could be tucked in ? After a fitful night, I rose about five-thirty, anxious to see Russia from ground level.

It was a twenty minute walk up the barren hill where I found several World War II redoubts that once housed guns pointing towards Russia. (During the war, the Russians took over the town. Many citizens escaped and lived for several years underground in the iron ore caves.) Remains of building foundations were scattered several hundred yards apart. I stared in the direction of Russia some ten to twelve miles away. What was over there ? The stark scene was endless miles of nothing but naked, stony little hills and valleys. There was a feeling of total desolation. There was no sign of civilization in any direction. On the wind swept hill my sweater and jacket did not provide enough warmth so I headed back down the hill into Kirkenes.

At 6:30 A.M. it looked like a well-maintained ghost town. No humans, no dogs, not even smoke coming out of chimneys. The mostly clapboard houses were all relatively small. Since there were no trees in sight, home construction materials (like virtually everything else to keep Kirkenes people alive) came by packet boat. This town, like dozens of others on the Norwegian west coast, survived through the once or twice weekly packet boat deliveries. I passed a green house, there a yellow, there a red one, there a tan one, just enough color to keep native spirits high in an otherwise colorless village.

The first person I saw was inside a circus tent just off a winding road at the edge of town. The man spoke English and told me he was part of a traveling carnival that once a year entertained the citizens with a few animals, some amusement rides, and fun and games. Another two days and they would be open for business. A few minutes later I was in the center of the town. It was reminiscent of a mid-western U.S. town, the kind with extra wide streets. There was an appliance store, a food store, a general store, a bank. At six-thirty in the morning not a soul was in sight. A hundred yards beyond the main street were the docks and a rocky shore front. I sat on a sea wall and peered out into the forbidding, frigid looking Artic Ocean.

Turning away from the cold wind, a man and woman responded to my "Good morning" with "Goot morneg." "Do you speak English?" I asked. Yes, they did. "Tell me about this church here by the sea. I understand the Germans shelled and destroyed the whole town in 1940. Is this the original church?" No, they said, it was rebuilt in 1959. It simply looked older.

Back on "Main Street," I noticed what looked like parking meters. Upon closer inspection, they turned out to be electrical outlets used to keep car engines warm and/or to help start them up in the extreme cold of winter. I remembered seeing similar devices in Fargo, North Dakota. Thus far on my walk I had seen no trees, no grass. Heading back on a different street I spotted green grass in front of one home with a few very small evergreen trees. Several other houses were similarly landscaped, some had green plants in their windows. A familiar satisfying smell hit my nostrils. I looked around and spotted smoke curling out of a chimney. Kirkenes was waking up.

Except for Hammerfest, a small town on an island just a bit northwest of Kirkenes, I had just walked from one end to the other of the second most northern town in Europe.

Before heading back up the hill to the hotel I came upon the village square with a small kiosk and bandstand in the center of the park. Next to it was a small bronze plaque memorializing the nineteen civilians killed by the Germans during the 1940 to 1945 period. It was a sobering end to an invigorating walk.

The three hundred foot packet boat Vesteraalen was our home for five days going from Kirkenes south along the coast to Bergen. The walking decks dead-ended fifty feet back of the ship's bow. My morning walks therefore required several about-faces and cross-deck cuts to make a lap. Nonetheless, those dead-ends were actually lifesavers for they momentarily kept me out of the biting North Sea wind. Heading towards the stern with the wind on my back would warm me up slightly before turning the corner to lean into the wind on the forward leg. All the while a diffused sun remained low and pale in the summer sky.

I peeked out my porthole on our second morning and saw we were approaching a dock. Dressing hurriedly I got on deck to watch our arrival in Tromso. I assumed we would be met by a tugboat with lots of men ashore ready to grab ropes. Instead, the ship coasted towards the dock and slowed to a standstill. Now parallel to the dock, the Vesteraalen suddenly thrust itself sideways using powerful jets of water spewing out of the ship's side. As it eased into the dock a single dockhand caught a small rope tossed to him from the stern. He then grabbed the heavier howser line attached to it and wrapped it around a large cleat. After he tied down one more rope from the bow we were docked. No tug, no dock crew, just one man. Easier than parking your car at the mall. I thought of the tugs and longshoremen it would have taken in New York Harbor.

Norwegian efficiency continued to impress me. A small forklift raced out of a warehouse towards us. A ten-foot-square panel door swung open from the side of the ship allowing a ramp to slide out on the dock. The forklift barely paused before scooting into the hold. Thirty-seconds later out it backed out carrying two huge crates. Spinning around on the dock, it raced back into the warehouse. Now there were two forklifts. The second barely paused for the first before it too scooted into the hold. As the process continued, the ship's elevator brought ever more crates and pallets to the exit level. The forklifts moved as tirelessly as worker bees unloading pollen from a flowering hedge. Twenty minutes later they were done. Now on the dock were crates of frozen shrimp, crabs and fish from Iceland and Greenland. The Norwegian fishing fleet, helped along by the Russians, had so over-fished the formerly rich Norwegian waters that these coastal towns had to import their seafood from a thousand miles away.

It was still only five-thirty in the morning as Polly Woodbridge and I walked up the hill into town along an empty street lined with stores. Tromso was a neat and tidy place totally rebuilt after the Nazis had left it in rubble. At the very top of the hill stood a steepled church painted a rich deep blue from top to bottom. It virtually glowed in the early light in an otherwise colorless neighborhood. The Vesteraalen would soon leave and would not, we knew, wait an instant for tardy passengers. For only a moment we sat on the top of the hill and looked back over the bay sparkling in the early morning sun. Cool. Quiet. Peaceful. Then we walked back briskly down the hill into Tromso, hailing the only Tromsonian we passed, and walked up the ramp just as the same single dockhand started to unwind the howser from the cleat to prepare the ship for departure. In 6 days the Vesteraalen made 11 stops, some times at night. The port turnaround time ranged from 30 to 90 minutes. Each time there was the same efficient loading and unloading of vital supplies for these isolated towns.

There were few early risers on subsequent mornings. The fifty passengers were distracted by hearty Norwegian breakfasts—sardines, cheeses, fresh fruits and compotes, rashers of bacon, boiled eggs nestled in a woven basket in the shape of a chicken, spiced meats, multi-shaped breads and rolls, jellies, American-style cereals, coffee, cocoa, juices. Knowing an early shipboard walk on a brisk morning would create an especially healthy appetite, I planned ahead by going an extra mile each day. It may not really have controlled my weight, but at least it let me self-indulge more freely.

The Hawksbury River estuary is forty miles north of Sydney, Australia. In March 1987 a brand new ship, the Lady Hawksworth, was commissioned. Princeton friends Ray and Betty Bowers, Jack and Nancy Worthington and Randy and I were lucky enough to book passage on her maiden voyage, a two-and-a-half day trip up and back to the mouth of the river at the Pacific Ocean.

On the morning after our first night on the Lady Hawksworth, I rose at six to walk around the deck of the 224 foot shallow-draft ship. As with many of these smaller boats, it was not possible to make a complete circuit around the main deck though the top deck provided me with a three hundred and sixty degree view. This day was a moving walk, emotionally and literally. The boat quietly whined its way silently up the bending river. Not a ripple was on it. Low fog enveloping the ship created an eerie glow as the rising sun ahead tried to penetrate. The reds and pinks were breathtaking. As the fog dispersed it permitted me a clearer view of the three hundred yard wide river.

There was thick undergrowth along the desolate shores and was no sign of life. A small house with a dock appeared, then nothing for miles. The next house was right at the water's edge with a huge palisade of rock behind it with no sign of a driveway nor of a road. How did people get there ? Did they boat up from Sydney? Were these only vacation homes? My reverie was abruptly interrupted by two water-skiers who roared by the ship and waved up at me.

I went down the steps to the lower deck and said good morning to two young crewmen painting the railings on the foredeck. "Morning, matey," replied the younger of the two with a thick Aussie accent. It was a unique mixture of English cockney and the drawl of an American southerner. They were students, new to ship life and working as deckhands during their summer vacations. Now, in March, their southern hemisphere summer was drawing to a close. They told me that many students need only to go through only the equivalent of the 10th grade to earn a certificate qualifying them for many kinds of jobs.

As my fortieth turn around the deck ended Jack and Ray came up the steps. Sadly for them, the sun had now burned off all of the fog. The vivid colors were gone. Still, the day was bright and clear and the heat was already starting to rise. The three of us hung over the railing to watch the sunlight dancing on the river, catching glimpses from time to time of civilization in an otherwise wild terrain. An hour later we landed near a settlement and traveled inland by bus to visit a horse ranch and historic inn built a hundred years before when Australia was much like the early U.S. "wild west." It still looked like unspoiled frontier land.

For the three months before I was born and for the first eight years of my life, my family spent summers in Ephraim, Wisconsin with a population—so noted a sign at each end of town—of one hundred and ninety-two souls. Ephraim was what our summers were all about. My brothers, our sister and I rejoiced in visiting our grandfather. With him we sputtered around in his speedboat affectionately called the Whoopee, fished with him at five in the morning, and learned how to swim at Sandy Beach.

Fifty years later when my brother Wells invited me to go sailing at Ephraim on a forty-foot sailboat he chartered, I jumped at the chance. We set off with his two sons who had never been sailing. Wells was an old salt, and had let me crew for him when we were teenagers. What could be more exciting than revisiting Ephraim and sailing at the same time? But, I asked myself, how would I be able to keep my morning walking streak going while being aboard a small sailboat ?

After a deep sleep, occasionally roused by the gentle rocking and lapping of the waves on the hull, I crept up to the deck as dawn brightened. Between our sloop and the small semi-circular island several hundred yards away were a dozen other small boats. As if guided by a tide, a small breeze had them all headed in the same direction. The absolute quiet was barely broken with the splash of a fish that jumped out of the water fifty feet away.

I eased into our small 8-foot long dory and quietly rowed ashore. Passing through a small field of unmown grass with many wild blueberry bushes, I remembered blueberry picking with Grandma and the subsequent reward of blueberry pancakes the next morning. Alas, these berries were still green.

Walking past vacation cottages nestled close to the water I realized something had been added during the last sixty years. The little island had telephone and electricity poles. What had not changed was the buzz and attack of mosquitos. Suddenly, swat! swat! They were still around. Back at the sandy and stony beach I sat on a boulder to savor the scene—the calm water, the gently rocking boats, the bluffs of Peninsula State Park and its lookout tower a mile away, and the village of Ephraim four miles across the water. That tower climb as a child had been a major effort. Was it 130 steps to the top? I remember being so proud making it all the way up with my 7-year-old legs. Now I would be just as proud to make it again with 60-year-old legs. Rowing back out to the sloop, I knew full well by this time Wells would be cooking up breakfast in the galley for us all.

That night we tied up at a dock, making the start of my walk the next morning an easy stride down the plank to shore. I strode past towering pine trees, past sleeping campers in their sleeping bags, past a couple making flapjacks and bacon on a grill over an open fire, and arrived at the foot of the one hundred foot tower lookout at Peninsula Park. Ten steps, a platform, ten steps, another platform, up I went. Eighty-eight steps later, I stood at the top. It wasn't 130 steps after all! Below me in all directions lay the treasured places of my childhood: Ephraim, Sandy Harbor, even Washington's Island, ten miles to the north. After absorbing the view, it was with a great sense of accomplishment I went down the 88 steps and returned to the sloop. My pedometer read three miles. It really should have read fifty years.

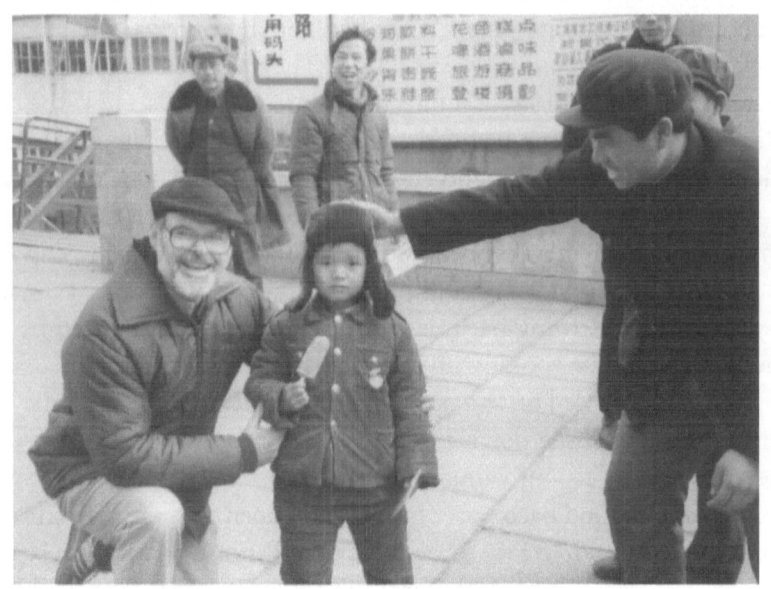

Making friends during pre-breakfast walk in Shanghai, China
March 15, 1985

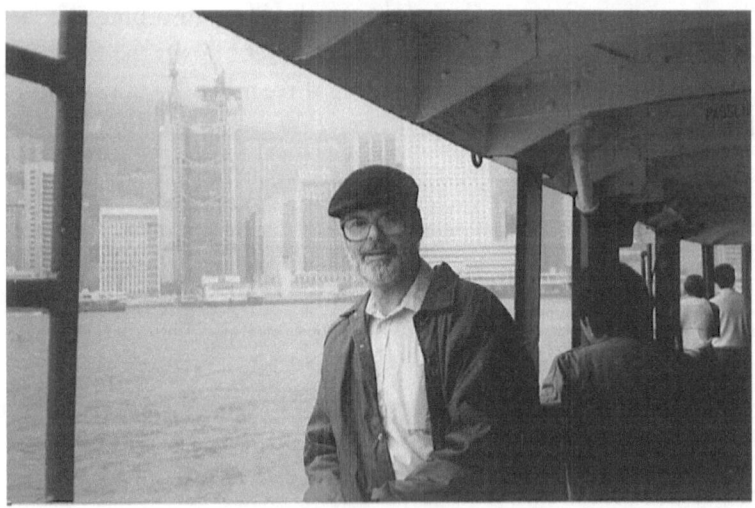

7 a.m. aboard the Kowloon-Hong Kong Star Ferry
March 7, 1985

CHAPTER 11

WALKS WHILE TRIPPING
AWAY FROM HOME

". . . success in walking is not to let your right foot know what your left foot doeth. Your heart must furnish such music that in keeping time to it your feet will carry you around the globe without knowing it."
—John Burroughs "The Exhilirations of the Road"

Early morning coastal fog covered the entire village of Corfe Castle. The magnificent ruins of the castle atop the hill overlooking the tiny town were invisible. It was my second visit to one of the most charming towns in England, and feeling I knew my way about notwithstanding the dense fog, I headed out of town.

I walked north past an inn, some cottages, a small school, and a new apartment development. A car appeared and disappeared in the fog. An unseen dog defending his masters' territory offered several warning barks. After 20 minutes I turned east on a crossroad assuming it must intersect another road heading south back into town. Sure enough, a few minutes later another road appeared. But was it the way home?

Ten minutes later my judgement proved wrong. It was the wrong road. Should I retrace my steps rather than get lost? The fog lifted just enough to reveal a field on my right. Perhaps crossing the field might be a shortcut back?

I was having a marvelous time not knowing exactly where I was. As I crossed the heath two grazing horses appeared out of the fog. They casually looked me over as three more horses appeared beyond. Suddenly out of the fog to my right a dog came walking just ahead of his leather booted master.

"If I continue across the field in this direction will I get back to the main road into town?" I asked.

"No," the man responded taking his pipe out of his mouth. Pointing his walking stick he said, "There's fencing in the direction you're going without any stiles. To get back to the main road you'll have to go over there past those horses. Won't you join me?"

Harry Pate introduced me to his Springer Spaniel, James, and the three of us walked towards the horses. Two continued to graze, two took off in a romp as the sun began to break up the fog. I took a deep breath to inhale the clean morning dampness and smell of grass. My new found guide with his walking cane, knickers, leather boots, pipe and dog walked off vigorously and disappeared into the fog. The scene was as English as anyone might concieve. Over my left shoulder the rising sun revealed the top of the Corfe Castle ruins. Moments later I was back at the Bankes Arms Inn in the center of the village. The sky was blue. The air was crisp. My walk had been more than I could possibly have expected.

The charm and variety of walks in England are second to none. Green hills and dales, streams and woods, thatched roofed houses and lovely gardens, hospitable people, everywhere gentle countryside, freedom to walk across pastures. I once had four very special walks in a row. We stayed at the White Hedge Country House in charming little Alfriston in Sussex south of London. Each of the 32 rooms were furnished with French period furniture by the Francophile owners. My morning walk took me through the village, past several shops, an old inn, the Clergy House, and the first old building in England to be put into the National Trust. The grass by the gently flowing river was especially green that morning. The next day we stayed at the Brickwall Hotel in Sedlescombe. Up the main road I went and turned into a long driveway leading uphill to I knew not where. Three hundred yards beyond a small school campus came into view. On the way back down I met three boys from Palestine who spoke English well enough to tell me they were students up the hill at the Petrozelli School, part of a refugee village.

The next morning in front of The White Lion Hotel in Tenterton, Kent there was an exceptionally broad street perhaps 100 feet wide. Between the curb and a row of stores on either side was an apron of well trimmed grass. As I passed a quaint church, my wife Randy came towards me as she headed out for her walk. We seldom walked together so I reversed my direction to join her. The next day we were at the Great Dane Hotel in Hollinghorse, also in Kent, perhaps a mile from the famous Leeds Castle which we were to see later that morning. I walked out in the rain, across a gateway bridge, and along the water which surrounded much of the castle. I stopped to say hello to a man who was standing by a horse and wagon capable of seating about a dozen people. It was open on all sides with a crude homemade roof over it. As we exchanged small talk, the horse was dejectedly hanging its head. After breakfast, when we returned for our formal tour, the wagon was now bumping along the road loaded with customers who had paid a premium so as not to take the long walk from the main road. As if it was proud of its job, this time the horse's head was high.

We were visiting Dorothy and Dick who had moved from Princeton to Hendersonville, N.C. During the October morning walk through rolling Carolina hills, I unexpectedly came upon a summer camp nestled among pine groves.

The mess hall door was open. Huge kitchen pots hung on the wall. I peeked into the nature lodge, took a quick look into the infirmary, and casually walked through the scrub pine grove down to the dock by a small lake. The mirror-like surface made perfect reflections of the trees along the shore. A dozen canoes were stacked on racks on the beach. My mind went back as an 11-year-old to Camp Winona in Denmark, Maine and to a reunion visit just two years before.

It had been a cool September morn. I made a quick decision not to dash into the lake for the traditional wake up skinny dip I'd enjoyed as a kid. It was memorable to walk through the pine grove, step into one of the tents (no cabins for real campers!), and visit the wiggy lodge we used so often for instruction, story telling, and singing. Up the hill I went to the old baseball field. At age 11 it had seemed like a long hike back down to the water's edge. Out on the dock I removed my shoes to test the water. I took a paddle, pulled a canoe into the water and gingerly stepped into the middle to push out from shore.

Thoughts of Camp Winona 60 years before faded as the beauty of the North Carolina lake shifted my mind back to yet another early lake memory.

I was back again in Ephraim, Wisconsin sixty years later as if no time had passed. There was Anderson's dock, "The BIG DOCK," where the lake steamers like the Carolina had docked and where Grandpa kept live bait. As a prank, my older brothers one night had painted "THIS DOCK UNSAFE" in three foot high letters on the roof of the dock's barn facing the village. Anderson's store at the water's edge used to have penny candy, licorice, and ice cream cones for a nickel. It was still there, now a living museum just as it had been 60 years before. Across the road and a hundred yards further was the riding stable. The several horses in the stalls had the same horsey smell. This was *MY* horse smell, the place where I first rode a horse at age 3. To scare me my brothers had told me his name was DYNAMITE, that he was the fastest horse in the world. I remember nervously saying "giddyup, Dynamite" much to the amusement, I am sure, of my elders.

On towards the little village I went past Grandpa's white stone house, the biggest house in the village. His lakeside artesian well had the coldest, freshest water I ever tasted. The road side of the house was where I had operated a lemonade stand one day. Grandpa helped me set up and Grandma had cooked fresh doughnuts all day long to keep up with the brisk sales my sister and I made. Five cents for a doughnut. Five cents for a glass of lemonade. My sister Ginny was 7 and I was 5. We must have made $3.00 that day.

The macadam road had been gravel 60 years before. I recalled the smell of fresh tar the road crews sprayed on to minimize the dust. I walked past the Pine Grove Hotel where we had stayed in a cottage across from Grandpa's house. Mr. Olsen, the owner, had taken me out at 5:30 am one time to the farm where with wonderment I helped him get fresh eggs right from under the chickens and milk cans of unpasteurized fresh milk. Mrs. Olsen showed me the big pots and pans in the kitchen where she made that especially good apple sauce.

Wilson's store was still there in the center of the village. What fun it had been to sit up on the stool to have a 10 cent soda, hamburgers for a nickel. Next door was the town theater—actually the town hall—where I saw my first movie. A woman had played the piano up front for the silent film. Those long benches were uncomfortable. The movie classic was WINGS with Richard Arlen. It had exciting World War I dogfights and biplane crashes created by stuntman Dick Grace. (Had he really broken every bone in his body over the years?)

It was now 8 am and I wasn't at Camp Winona in Maine or at my grandfather's in Ephraim, Wisconsin. I was surrounded by pine trees, by a lake, in a winterized camp site in Hendersonville, North Carolina. It had stimulated special memories and it was time for breakfast a mile away with my hosts.

My brother Ed often joined his Princeton '39 classmates to attend the Princeton-Dartmouth football game in Hanover, New Hampshire. Never before had he invited me to join him so I suspected nothing. Friday night while we were having cocktails at the Woodstock Inn a few miles from Hanover I understood why he had invited me. One by one my four children and their spouses walked in to surprise me on my 65th birthday. My 94-year-old mother arrived. I had just dropped her off the night before in Connecticut presumably to spend the weekend with my daughter Mary. Finally my brother Wells and his wife Jean arrived from St. Louis. A marvelous surprise had been orchestrated by my wife who had kept it a secret for months.

It began with all thirteen of us retiring to a reception room where with due love and great planning and execution they presented me with mementos of my life wrapped up in creative and sometimes corny and occasionally impertinent verses. A photo at age 4 in my scratchy woolen bathing suit—school graduation—group family pictures—a narrative about my broadcasting career.

Ed Hitz, the NBC-TV sales manager who hired me to start the day the NBC-Television Network was formed on December 1, 1949, had assigned me to the Lucky Strike advertising agency. They needed a studio for a major new one hour show, the debut of the first Hollywood star to regularly perform on TV—"Robert Montgomery Presents." Opening night Bob Hope was among the important people who came to the famous "21" for a post show reception I was asked to arrange. Thereafter on rehearsal break I occasionally had lunch with Bob Montgomery in the Rainbow Room.

As one of the five original NBC-TV network salesman, I obtained advertisers for the Sid Caesar "Show of Shows," the "Garroway at Large" show, "Kukla, Fran and Ollie," the first advertiser on the "Today Show," Kate Smith on daytime and then night time TV, and "Four Star Revue" featuring Jimmy Durante alternating with Jack Carson, Danny Thomas and Ed Wynn. After the opening Ed Wynn show two twenty-seven year-olds–an agency executive named Dave Mahony and I–followed Wynn from one nightclub to another until 5 am.

TV was new, exciting, expensive. Everything was a first, everything was live. It was seven years before videotape and it was exciting becoming friends with many of the TV stars. Nineteen cities could see live television. Less than 1½ million people had TV sets. Every week new cities would be added to the expanding network and hundreds of thousands were buying sets as prices came down.

Thanks to being involved in the media in years to come I was to meet Herbert Hoover, Presidential candidate Sen. Jack Kennedy and his brother Bobby, former President Harry Truman, presidential candidate Richard Nixon, Eleanor Roosevelt, Presidents Eisenhower, Ford, Reagan and Vice President Bush. I am sure each of them forgot me a minute later, but for me it was memorable, an always stimulating, always exciting career and some of it was now being replayed for me.

It had been raining hard when we arrived in Woodstock that Friday evening making Saturday morning wet and cloudy. Still, the gorgeous fall colors were everywhere as I set out for my morning walk. Armed with my umbrella and rubbers I took off to explore the village, headed west past the village green, then reversed my direction to pass a variety of small stores. I spotted a New England rarity, an old covered bridge. Walking through the restored bridge brought back cherished memories of others I had seen as a young boy traveling through New Hampshire and Vermont. What fun it had been driving through and hearing mother say "duck your head!" and stopping to permit horse and buggies to clip-clop over the wooden flooring. I recalled paddling down the Saco River as a summer camper and passing under similar bridges. Now my walk through the barn-like structure to the other side was slow and deliberate to relish every step.

Several school children waiting for their bus returned my smile. A few raindrops prompted me to step back under the bridge. Not knowing when I might ever again pass through a real covered bridge again I turned and walked through the bridge a second time. Little had my family known when they arranged the surprise birthday gathering that they would provide me with such a memorable birthday walk.

The six hour drive from Princeton landed the President of the American Boychoir School John Ellis and me in Manchester, Vermont at 9 pm. The Inn at Manchester was a charming old home that had been converted into a bed and breakfast. There was still enough light to see the mountain above the town and I looked forward eagerly to my New England walk the next morning.

The sun woke me at 5 :30. After 20 minutes of luxuriating in a comfortable bed, I unlocked the front door and stepped into a 58 degree slightly overcast morning. The grass was wet and I inhaled deeply for the air smelled crisp and fresh.

Why I turned to the right instead of the left I do not know. Happily it was the right decision for a perfect walk. A hundred yards up Main Street was a private home displaying a lawyer's shingle. Three houses beyond was another lawyer's signpost.

I passed the 1811 house, a well preserved old Inn. Just beyond was the broad main street with clapboard houses and shops on either side. I had not yet seen a human being nor a car when I spotted two Japanese gentlemen closely inspecting historical markers. Their presence in this 18 century village somehow seemed incongruous. We bowed and smiled at each other.

On the left was the high steepled Congregational Church, on the right the huge Equinox Hotel which stretched the better part of an entire block. It obviously was a vintage building so I walked into the lobby. It was like walking into 1900. To the right off the large turn-of-the-century furnished lobby was a breakfast room, a lounge to the left. Big stuffed chairs, a big stone fireplace. The National Register of Historic Places plaque was prominently displayed by the front door. I subsequently learned the Equinox had once been *THE* place to come for summer vacations, seminars and conventions. New owners were planning to once again make it prominent.

Down Main Street I continued past St. Paul's Catholic Chapel, past the Johnny Appleseed Book Store and past one large house after another, all with big front porches, and a few with swinging benches. Many houses displayed American flags, all the lawns were freshly cut, hanging on several front doors were flower baskets. A woman's straw hat hung on another. Each house looked freshly painted, one with a bright red front door. A one floor long yellow house looked like it could be the oldest in town and feeling like a trespasser, I walked up to the front door. Sure enough, it had an Historic Places plaque. In the backyard of the next house was a hammock and a small screened-in kiosk-type structure with a child's table and four chairs.

It was now 6:30 and still no sign of people or cars. At the edge of town I started to turn up towards the mountain when a sign caught my attention: "Ekwanok Golf Club, Private." Surely no one would mind my walking down the club drive at this time of day. A few minutes later I stood by the club house and first tee. By the ball washer was a 16 inch high bronze golfer statuette poised to drive. The grass on the green was as green and manicured as any I had ever seen. The adjoining fairway was beautifully cropped. Stretching out across a valley between the club house and a mountain several miles away were damp fairways and greens beginning to be bathed with sunlight. My own footprints on the wet grass caught my attention as I turned back.

A cluster of white birch trees to the left of the fairway recalled fond memories. I've loved white birches ever since I was introduced to them in Wisconsin by Grandpa when I was four. He taught me how to strip small portions of birch bark to make napkin rings and post cards.

On the way back I passed The American Museum of Fly Catching, "Open 10-3, Monday-Friday." Would that my expert fishing grandson Chris could be with me to go through it. Back at the Manchester Inn John Ellis was sitting on the front porch. A quick report on my walk persuaded him to join me in the car so he too could see and enjoy some of what I had just seen. We returned promptly at 7 to have a full "Farmers Breakfast" served by the owners family style with other over-nighters. It was an appropriate finale to a peaceful morning walk in a town that was the quintessence of all New England villages.

For my 60th birthday we decided to live it up with a trip to London by reserving a room at the famous Savoy Hotel. On the morning of my big day I headed out to see some famous London sights. 500 feet from the Savoy Hotel is the Savoy Theatre on the Strand, probably the shortest and definitely the only street in Britain where they drive on the right (to conveniently let off passengers in front of the Theater and the hotel). Off through history I walked to see English classic landmarks—Parliament and Westminster Abbey by the Thames, St. James Park, and Buckingham Palace. Four miles later, having savored every step of my birthday walk, room service provided a tasty full English breakfast fit for a king and queen. As we sat down, the waiter opened up the French windows of our room so we might also digest the view of the tree-lined Thames River below. It was an incomparable beginning of my out-of-the-ordinary birthday.

Christmas at the Plaza in New York? What could be more elegant! We were without Christmas plans nor did Jack and Nancy have plans. So, for a few days together we did it up royally in New York City—theater, dining out, walking up and down Fifth Avenue and window shopping. While lunching at the Renaissance Restaurant by the ice skating rink in Rockefeller Center we watched youngsters, oldsters, and show-offs skate round and round. Above us was the Center's annual huge lighted Christmas tree.

We all decided it would be fun the next day to have breakfast downtown atop the World Trade Center overlooking lower Manhattan, the Battery and the Statue of Liberty. It was a cool morning the day before Christmas when Jack and I left the Plaza at 5th Avenue and 59th Street in our walking shoes. At 7 am we headed south for the six miles to our destination. Our wives were to take a taxi an hour later to met us. Fifth Avenue was almost devoid of people when we started and auto fumes had yet to permeate the air. Downhill past St. Patrick's Cathedral we went to catch a fleeting view of Rockefeller Plaza, eased our pace past stores to glimpse the beautiful store window nativity scenes, continued downhill past Abercrombie and Fitch, jewelry stores, leather shops, Brooks Brothers, across an uncrowded 42nd Street intersection, by the huge New York Public Library and past the Empire State Building.

The elegance of 5th Avenue between 55th and 40th street began to fade as we hit 30th street. Right down the middle of an empty 5th Avenue we continued to the famous Washington Square with its miniature Arc de Triomphe, then past the big Metropolitan Life Insurance headquarters across the park. Jack pointed out the Mews (named after London mews I assumed) where he had once lived. Next came junk stores, ethnic restaurants and finally Chinatown. After a leisurely 1 hour and 40 minute walk we arrived in the Wall Street area with its towering modern buildings, walked by the old AT&T building and arrived at the huge World Trade Towers Plaza whose main floor starts one flight up from the street. The 107 story twin tower building glittered in the morning light. 90 seconds later the elevator delivered us a quarter of a mile up to the Window on the World restaurant on the top floor. We took a table for four immediately adjacent to a window just as Randy and Nancy arrived after their 25 minute taxi ride.

My chair, inches from the outside window, permitted me to look straight down—1000 feet below! Beyond was a breathtaking view of New York Harbor and in motion was the Staten Island Ferry and two ocean-going merchant vessels. The breakfast and the view capped an exhilarating one-of-a-kind six mile walking experience down the middle of 5th Avenue.

The airport Hilton in Detroit sits right by the terminal. For my morning walk I knew I'd find no country lanes, no city streets. The night before I asked myself—where could I walk? The next morning was a bitterly cold winter day. The wailing sounds of jet engines warming up echoed throughout the area as I went out the front door. A few cars and taxis buzzed by. Sure enough, the sidewalk ended after a few hundred yards leaving only some grass on which to safely walk.

I crossed what would be a busy road in another hour and headed down the street to stop behind a high wire-meshed fence a hundred feet from several 747's. Standing there and taking in the scope of these planes was impressive. They are BIG. Several men were washing down an American Airlines plane as mechanics were working on another. I could see the name of several of the planes written on the fuselage up near the pilot's window. Standing this close to the flight-line watching ground crew maintenance brought into focus other days when ground crews were making last minute checks before my B-29 training and combat missions.

Cloud cover below and 150 mph jet stream winds at 25,000 feet over Japan was causing inaccurate bombing. Little did any of us know what General LeMay was planning until a mission briefing the afternoon of March 9, 1945.

All of the 9th Bomb Group crews were there for a maximum effort. With Col. Eisenhart announcing the mission would be flown at night at 5500 feet, concerned murmuring was heard throughout the briefing hall. Then the intelligence officer could not confirm or deny the possible presence of Japanese barrage balloons hanging over Tokyo. "You'll find out when you get there," he said. More concerned murmuring. The weather officer reported cloud cover the entire 1500 miles up to Japan and back to Tinian—no chance of me using necessary celestial navigation. The gunnery officer got up and announced that no 50 caliber bullets would be on board for any of the 10 guns. "You'll be coming in at 5500 feet, Saipan at 6000 feet, Guam at 6500 feet on individual sorties at 2 am—you may think other B-29's are enemy fighters and shoot at them. Further, the reduced weight will permit us to carry more bombs." 48 crews loudly groaned and looked at each other almost in disbelief. Survival of this mission seemed like a long shot. The briefing broke up and we returned to our tents. Perhaps like many others I wrote a letter to my bride of 11 months telling her of my love and counseling her to remarry if I should not come back. Like many others, my letter was conditionally deposited with the 1st squadron's operation officer for mailing—just in case.

About 7 P.M. dozens and dozens of B-29's were taxiing from their pads to the head of three runways. It was an impressive, awe inspiring sight. Simultaneously B-29's on parallel runways headed down the 6000 foot runways each loaded with 7000 gallons of gas and 7000 pounds of incendiary bombs. It had not been a pretty sight a few days before when a loaded B-29 crashed on take-off. As we took off to the northeast we could see two B-29's simultaneously taking off on Saipan runways several miles away.

The sun was fading as 314 airplanes from Tinian, Saipan and Guam 120 miles to the south headed north towards Japan. To conserve gas each plane was flying at 1000 feet en route on its individual sortie. Using dead reckoning from 12-hour old weather information, I set the course for Lloyd Welken my airplane commander. (The "old" man was 23.) But was I on course? I popped in another stay-awake pill in anticipation of a 15-hour mission. (Everyone except the navigator had chances for a nap.) There a mile to the left and to the right were other planes all heading in slightly different northern directions. Seven hours later my ETA (estimated time of arrival) indicated Tokyo should have been in sight. Thoburn, the co-pilot reported nothing in view. Through the intercom Gregg, the flight engineer said "Herb, if you don't find Tokyo within a half hour we won't have enough gas to get back to Tinian."

Guessing perhaps we'd flown too far north, we headed west to intercept the coast of Japan. Another 10 minutes and no Japan.

Could headwinds have caused us to be further south? "Head north," I said. A minute later, Bombardier Bill Flaherty, our impish 5 foot 6 Irishman from Massachusetts, said "I see a huge glow in the sky dead ahead." We started to climb from 1000 to 5000 feet to arrive over Tokyo about 2 am. Most of the 300 planes had preceded us having created an incredible fire storm. We could clearly see the Emperors Palace we had been told to avoid. Our dark glasses diffused the roaming searchlights from below. All of us were wearing heavy chest flak suits, though some of us had put the flak helmet in the crotch area to protect "the family jewels." A mortally wounded B-29 off to the right headed slowly down into the fire storm as Flaherty let the bombs go in an area not yet in total flames.

"Let's get out of here" someone yelled as Lloyd swung east and raced the air speed up to 300. A few minutes later we were safely over the ocean heading south when more flak suddenly exploded in the sky from flak barges below. An easy turn of the ship took us out of harms way. Off came the flak suits, cigarettes were lit and everyone reached for sandwiches and coffee. Unlike other World War II airplanes, the B-29 was the first pressurized plane, had radar and Loran, semi-computerized remote gun control, even a cot in the rear section for naps during the 13 to 16 hour missions.

Four hours later I asked Snowden, the radar operator, to turn on the equipment to pick up Pajaros, the northern most Mariannas Island and instructed him to follow the islands and bring us home. Exhausted and without sleep for almost 24 hours I crawled into the tunnel connecting fore and aft of the plane and fell asleep. Twenty minutes later Radio Operator Phillips woke me to announce "we are lost!" Now with a clear sky, I took a quick fix on the now available north star from the navigators plastic dome and crossed with a reverse direction radio signal from Tinian to re-establish our position. We landed 14 hours and fifty minutes after take-off with five minutes of gas left. Fourteen of the 314 planes—154 men—had been lost in that annihilating raid.

Our crew flew on four of the five fire raids during that ten day period first over Tokyo, then Nagoyga, Osaka, Kobe and a return to Nagoyga. The devastation of each city was enormous with only seven B-29's lost in the other four raids. We heard something like 15 square miles of Tokyo had been burned out but it was not until April 1957 in a San Diego newspaper that I read all the details starting with the headline: "Raid on Tokyo Deadliest in Annals of War," ". . . not as devastating were the A Bomb attacks on Hiroshima and Nagasaki, nor any single raid on Berlin, Hamburg, or Dresden . . . 15.8 densely populated square miles were consumed in a fire storm so intense that no debris was left . . . 267,171 buildings destroyed, about one fourth of Tokyo . . . 83,793 dead, 40,918 wounded, 1,008,005 persons rendered homeless." Gen. Laurance Kuter who had written an article on the raid said it "became evident to the Japanese capitol that the war was lost."

The memory of that particular mission must have remained vivid in every B-29 flyer ever since. To the Japanese—even those not yet born—the date March 10, 1945 is a date remembered along with the atomic bomb dates of August 6th and August 9th of Hiroshima and Nagasaki.

The whining start-up noise of the huge American Airlines 747 in front of me at the Detroit Airport snapped me out of my reminiscing. The now almost deafening sound of jet engines warming up encouraged me to move rapidly to reach the virtually empty American Airlines building.

The open spaces of an airport makes winter winds particularly cold and the indoor interlude helped warm my freezing ears. Outdoors again, I watched Marriott catering trucks unloading breakfast meals for two planes. Whatever the menu, one thing I knew for sure, the passengers would have hunger pangs for at least an hour after take-off. Why can't they serve pre-cooked meals sooner?

A cold hour had passed since leaving the Hilton. There had been no countryside, no trees, no birds, no dogs, no paths—just concrete, macadam, lots of buildings and noise. It had not been a likely place for a walk but it had generated powerful memories.

Guilin, often called China's most beautiful city, is also famous for its winding Lijiang River surrounded by hundreds of spectacular high pointed hills made of karst limestone (native to China and Yugoslavia). Our five hour trip downstream on a flat bottom boat was one of serene scenic splendor. As we passed one cone shaped hill, another shadowy one would be behind it. Then another and another—seemingly ad infinitum. As the boat floated downstream, there had been no sign of civilization when our guide spotted a grass hut and a man and woman working in a field. The boat was poled to the rivers edge. Twenty-five westerners stepped ashore into a beautiful but isolated Chinese back country. Would the couple resent our intrusion? The language barrier was graciously overcome by their nodding and smiling as they escorted us to their crude hut. It had no electricity, no running water, no toilets. It was just a shack in the wilderness. Still, inside was a pendulum clock along side photographs of their family. Many of us had our pictures taken with them to memorialize an unexpected rare encounter.

Back aboard our boat, the Chinese guides poled us into midstream as cooks began preparing a hot meal on the stern. Floating with the current we passed a small open boat with two fisherman tethering two cormorants thirty feet further out in the water. The birds dive for fish but since they have a rope tied around their necks they cannot swallow. The cormorants thus become fishermen for the fishermen.

A live fire on the rear deck heated large pots into which all kinds of raw foods were tossed. While waiting for our meal, I found the "toilet" facilities. It was a round hole in the bottom of the boat with river water sloshing through. There was no seat. In order to keep one's feet out of the sloshing water there was a shoe size block of wood on either side of the hole to place one's feet. Standing or squatting was a precarious experience.

Fixed position wooden seats faced fore and aft throughout the 35 foot long barge with a crude wooden table in between for dining purposes. A "hot pot" was brought to each table. Hot pots are perhaps 12 inches across and 7 to 8 inches deep. They look like an angel food cake pan. Filled with hot water, the water continues to boil thanks to a 3-5 inch diameter hole in the middle containing a hot charcoal fire. Raw vegetables, chicken, raw fish, mushrooms and some fat was brought to each table. Each of us then dipped our chopsticks into the boiling mass of food and pulled out our hot lunch. The food was very tasty and was washed down with excellent Tsing Tao Chinese beer. Dessert was fresh pineapple.

Six hours down the river we shopped at our termination point, the little village of Yangshuo and were returned to Guilin by bus over a yet to be finished road. Bumpity, bump, bump all the way back for over an hour. Toot, toot went our horn constantly warning nonchalant bicyclists, walkers, buffalos and pigs. Here, as elsewhere in China, we considered it a miracle busses did not hit any one.

The Li River excursion was the highlight of our visit to China. It had been a glorious day and I looked forward to my morning walk next day. We were to leave early so I started out at 6 am.

The front door of the Ronghu Hotel at Banyan Lake in Guilin was locked. I faced a new experience: I couldn't get out to walk! After walking around the lobby for 15 minutes a Chinese woman coming to work opened the door. With the sun not yet up, a huge 800 year old banyan tree by the road loomed like a monster in the dark. There were no street lights as I cautiously walked along Banyan Lake to the town's main street. Two little coffee shops were open. Six or eight men were seated at a counter while several more were sitting at a small sidewalk table. Cigarettes were being heavily puffed and deeply inhaled in what obviously was a daily ritual.

Around the corner and on a side street, a most trim and physical man about 35 was teaching his 12 to 13 year old daughter Kung Fu. "Yeow! Ugh! Zow!" he yelled. Facing each other, he brandished a sword left and right, as she side-stepped each attack. He dropped the sword and switched to attacking with his legs which shot up and out with lightning speed. Seeing it on television was one thing, but this was real in the real China.

The sun was almost up as my return route took me back along Banyan Lake when I heard Chinese music. There, 200 feet out in the middle of a little lake, was a tiny island connected to the shore by a winding wooden bridge. I walked out the 150 feet to the island to see 10 women doing Tai Chi in the middle of a small grove of trees. Meditative Tai Chi may not build muscles but the slow moving, graceful exercise is part of the Chinese culture. Moving in unison, the women were listening to the national

Chinese radio which not only provided music but Tai Chi instructions. Subsequently I found out that millions of other Chinese throughout the country simultaneously listen and do Tai Chi early each morning.

Later in the day I would not have seen the coffee shops, the Kung Fu, the Tai Chi. The early morning walk made the difference.

Every few years broadcasters held their annual convention in Dallas. Needing directions for my walk, some blocks away from the hotel I approached a policeman standing in front of a bank. As I got closer I realized it was a cast bronze figure. Could it be one of Princeton's own Seward Johnson's? The life-like policeman was holding a clearly readable bronze parking ticket in his hand. Sure enough, at the top it read "Princeton Township." Just beyond was a real policeman who told me how to get to the site where Lee Harvey Oswald had assassinated President Kennedy. Eight or nine blocks later I stood in a small park with a direct view up to the Book Repository building. I imagined the cavalcade passing by, shots ringing out, Mrs. Kennedy leaning over the President, the car disappearing under the railroad tracks. The historical marker placed nearby briefly states what had happened that November day in 1963. Across the road I noticed an unusual large semi-enclosed circular concrete structure. It turned out to be a simple open air monument and tribute to the late President. The rest of the walk was necessarily inconsequential.

My niece Ruth had been married the afternoon before in Glenview, Illinois. My brother arranged for Randy and me to stay at an old friend's house several miles away in Jack Benny's hometown of Winnetka. This Sunday morning was threatening and cool as I took note of my hosts address and headed out to where I did not know. Down one residential street I went, past a lot of well-to-do homes, turned left and stopped to jot names of the first two streets to help me find my way back. Ten minutes later on a broad avenue along Lake Michigan it began to rain as I went up hill past a sturdy stone block Episcopal church. The sexton was opening up the front door in anticipation of early service parishioners. Diagonally across the street was a large house with closed black iron gates blocking access to the two driveway entrances. Atop the tall gate post was a small vidicon camera. Obviously the owner had to be of considerable means not only to own such a large home but also to be so concerned with security. Subsequently I found out it belonged to Clement Stone, one of America's wealthiest men who had made a fortune in the insurance business.

A half mile beyond I went down an unpaved road to Lake Michigan. The beach was stony, sandy, and uninteresting. By now the rain had become a storm. I walked out to the end of a long dock in a torrent of wind and rain to look back at the shoreline. My umbrella was useless as it inverted itself in the wind. It was a scene of pounding waves, black clouds, and pelting rain.

Twenty minutes later near the railroad tracks a small convenience store was open that provided me shelter from the rain. The elderly owner was obviously a seven-day-a-week Old Mr. Reliable. I felt guilty imposing on the warmth of his store and bought a pack of gum.

Once again out in the rain I continued through the village until recognizing the name of a cross street I had jotted down. Ten minutes later at 8:30 am I was greeted by my hostess with a cup of coffee and appropriately for a Sunday . . . hot cross buns!

Mary, Queen of Scots, had slept in one part of the castle, the Earl of Bothwell in another with a secret passage connecting the two rooms. This was tantalizing enough history for us to advance book an overnight stay at Borthwick Castle twelve miles south of Edinburgh.

A small parking area was at the top of the steep drive up to the small twin-towered castle. As we arrived a slightly built young man in a dark suit was already walking across the drawbridge over the moat.

"You're the Hoblers, I presume" Peter said. Only later when we found ourselves to be the only overnight visitors did we understand how he knew. He took us into a huge room, fifty feet long, 24 feet wide with a 40 foot high cathedral ceiling. This Great Hall featured huge fireplaces at either end. Each was twenty feet across and 8 feet high. A small friendly fire was burning in one. Sparsely furnished with a few leather chairs, a sofa, coffee table and a rug, the room otherwise was empty except for a black table adorned with two candles. The dinner settings were set just for the two of us. Several large lances, medieval axes, and a variety of battle gear from the period were hung on the thick stone walls.

Carrying our bags, Peter took us up round and round the stone spiral staircase to the second floor, past the balcony overlooking the Great Hall (where once madrigal singers entertained), and through a slightly smaller version of the Great Hall to one of the 12 bedrooms. Ours was the Earl of Bothwell's bedroom. The outside wall was at least 3 feet thick of solid stone. Our window was an 8x12 inch archer's slit once used by crossbowmen for defense. Next to the huge double bed with its large oak beam posters and canopy stood the largest wardrobe cabinet I had ever seen. This armoire stood 8 feet tall by 8 feet wide. A single wooden chair was near the entrance to a 3x3 foot cubby hole, a former guard chamber, now converted into a bathroom.

We found our way back to the Great Hall to find an unexpected arrival, a Princeton classmate who we had left with other classmates some hours before at Ardsheal House 150 miles away. The three of us had an elegant dinner, cooked and served by the sole employee—Peter the doorman, Peter the manager, Peter the bellhop, Peter the maitre di and Peter the historian who told us all about Borthwick's history. That night as we slept in the Earl of Borthwick's bedroom we fantasized how he and his lover Mary Queen of Scots had secreted themselves in this small castle. And how did 5'10" Mary escape capture by lowering herself on a rope after squeezing out of one of those small windows? To add to the eerie atmosphere of our castle visit, all night long there was an unearthly whine of the wind outside the little window of our unheated stone room.

Could my morning walk provide me a medieval adventure? The road around the castle was about two miles long. Always keeping the castle in sight, I concluded I should constantly be alert for horses and attacking knights, for boiling oil being poured down upon them, and flumes of arrows flying through the air. But no such luck! At the end of the road I got within a hundred yards of the castle to find an impassable roaring stream between me and what I had anticipated would be the end of my walk. Seeing no bridge, I had to retrace my steps the same two miles, this time noticing a large indentation on one side of the castle. Peter subsequently explained it was due to canon fire in a long ago battle.

Near the castle in the village of Borthwick was an old church. I inspected some of its cemetery headstones dating back 150-200 years before returning to the castle. During an otherwise uneventful walk, I had tried to transplant myself back 400 years as I rounded the castle. I had my fantasies during my walk. Still, I had slept in it, right there in Lord Bothwell's chambers with my own Mary (whose nickname is Randy).

As Chairman of the American Boychoir School for 15 years, I had dreamed of the day that our choir might appear on the Boston Pops TV Christmas Show. The invitation finally came for December 19, 1989.

Thanks to having seen PBS Boston Pops concerts, the scene was very familiar. It was a thrilling experience to sit with hundreds of others at tables on the concert hall floor, watching Conductor John Williams and

following the TV cameras as the show was videotaped. John Williams'
gracious introduction to "America's foremost boychoir and one of the
world's finest" was followed by the 26 voice choir performing two numbers.
One was a touching duet by 12-year-old Evan Weber and noted opera
singer Barbara Hendricks. The audience response was thunderous and the
applause sustained. Actor Ed Asner narrated the story of "Yes, Virginia
there is a Santa Claus." Afterwards I joined the boys backstage to meet the
principals. It would be a year before millions would see the "Christmas at
the Pops" show on public television.

My thoughtful travel agent daughter Nancy had booked me into the
Copley Plaza because she reminded me that "Grampie and Grammie were
there on their honeymoon in 1914." As I checked in I tried to imagine my
parents checking in the same lobby 75 years before.

"Do you happen to have a record of registrations for March 1914?"
I asked. The young woman behind the counter looked at me with
astonishment.

"No, I'm sure we don't, Mr. Hobler, but if you will stop by in the
morning and ask the Manager he might know." Subsequently the Manager
confirmed no such records still existed.

At 6:30 am I asked for directions to the waterfront, and headed out
into a cold and windy morning. With my mind full of Boston's history,
its fabled "propriety," "Indians" and tea parties, Saltonstalls, Kennedys,
Lodges, Harvard and MIT I went downhill to Boston Harbor to find
Quincy Market.

The doors to the vast covered market place were open. Inside what
once were wharf warehouses were dozens of little shops. The renovation
of the building had been a major downtown urban project designed to
recapture an 18th and 19th century appearance. A few people were walking
inside the wide and long interior center aisle. A bakery was serving coffee
and muffins and fruit shops were catering to early risers and commuters.

I walked along the waterfront to the newly built Rose Wharf Hotel
where the night before I had arrived by ferry boat after an 8 minute ride
from Logan Airport. I wandered through the hotel lobby, picked up a
Boston Globe and headed back up hill to the Copley Plaza.

While most of the Copley Plaza had been renovated and the old
elegance replaced with more contemporary architecture, when I entered
the breakfast room I finally felt I could share a common experience with
my parents. It could not have changed in 75 years for it still had high

ceilings, paintings, sketches and photographs of the early 1900's (in old frames), a bookcase with well worn covers, and period tables and chairs. It must have looked exactly the same way when mother and dad had breakfast there a day or two after their March 30th, 1914 wedding in Illinois. I ate my breakfast quietly contemplating that day so many years before.

Professor of French at Rutgers University and Princeton classmate Reg Bishop and his wife Alice were guiding us through France for two weeks. He chauffeured us, dispensed money, ordered the right wine and foods, spoke the language and always found memorable overnight accommodations. At Le Mouin des Ruats, an inn a mile from the village of Avallon, we heard the babbling sound of a small waterfall all night as the waters of the small Le Cousin River passed just below our window.

The weather next morning was just cool enough for a light sweater. I walked up stream perhaps a half mile to find a footbridge to the other side pausing a few moments to watch the clear water below passing swiftly under the bridge. Slightly downstream was a small waterfall. I stepped down from the narrow bridge to begin a downstream walk along an infrequently used path that hugged the edge of the stream. For 45 minutes I stepped over boulders, roots, and stones, stooping from time to time to duck under thornbushes and tree limbs. The path was far from level, with numerous short up and down inclines. It was no place for a jogger. Except for the murmering of the brook and an occasional twittering of birds, the walk was peaceful and quiet. Here and there the early morning sun light filtered through the trees. Frequent patches of green moss on the trees confirmed the sun was seldom welcomed.

Two empty packs of cigarettes on the trail caught my eye. Marlboros and Camels. What thoughtless Americans had desecrated this trail? Only later did I find the heavy smoking French favored American cigarettes. The end of the trail seemed at hand when a stone bridge appeared ahead. Seeing no other exit from the trail, I opened a gate into the back yard of a private home and shortly found myself on the main street of the village of Avallon. Excepting for the barking of a dog, the village was asleep.

A group of Frenchmen came out of the town's only hotel to board a bus. Just beyond in an alley lay a very old and unperturbed dog. He lifted one eyebrow at me. A Citroen went by and then the petite tin lizzy of all time, a Deux Cheveau. I stopped to look at a decrepit unoccupied stone house. Two shutters were gone, one was hanging by a thread, the splintered front door was half open, and an upstairs window was broken. Contrarily, next to it was a small, well-maintained house with pretty flowers in a window box. Like so many French houses, it too was made of stone, had a drab color and typically closed, unpainted shutters.

There was little more to the town so I crossed a bridge to head back upstream along a narrow two lane road. A large clearing strewn with new mown hay smelled delicious. Three large ducks waddled across a farmers field. Two donkeys munched hay in a trough.

Except for those few minutes in the village, I had felt totally isolated from the world for over an hour. Not even a car passed me during my twenty-five minute return. I had discovered a walk of abundant beauty and serenity. I was even ready for the daily, always the same French breakfast of croissants, rolls, jams and cheese.

300 of my first 3000 walking days were away from home: the charming village of Corfe Castle in Dorset, England with castle ruins atop a small hill and the Golden Retriever and cat side-by-side in a second story window in the village . . . Alice Springs in the desolate middle of Australia and walking the sandy new 9 hole golf course there that had recently been dedicated by Greg Norman . . . the mornings along the Kuaui shores when we visited the Worthington's in Hawaii's garden island . . . Bergen, Norway along the wharves and up the hill by colorful houses . . . London along the Thames and past Buckingham Palace . . . St. Louis looking for golf balls at the nearby St. Louis Country Club and Tucson, Arizona for a WWII B-29 reunion when, while walking through cactus fields I met a woman with a small dog who knew my friend J. Merrill Knapp in Princeton.

In Beijing there was the rising sun reflecting on the shiny aluminum siding of the Great Wall Hotel . . . the Tokyo experience of finding a park at 6:30 am two blocks from my daughter's apartment just as 50 men and women started exercising to a national wake-up radio show blaring out on speakers (resulting in my joining them each morning thereafter for five days) . . . walks each morning along the Estoril coast in Portugal and accidentally catching an early morning fish auction . . . the spectacular sunrise and moonset behind the Alhambra in Grenada, Spain with the view looking down on the city and off into the mountains.

The walk up and down hills in Oakland, California while visiting my nephew Dave Hobler . . . the many morning walks from daughter Debbie's house in Santa Barbara down into town from their hilltop home as well as walks in the opposite direction up into California foothills being bathed by the early morning sun . . . walking from the Sheraton Hotel adjoining the Universal lot in Los Angeles up the hill and looking down into the back lot to see Hollywood sets with false fronts . . . wandering through the beautifully maintained cemetery in Casnovia, New York the morning of the Princeton-Colgate football game hoping to find a Hobler ancestor.

And, finally, that chance encounter and conversation in Santa Barbara with an attractive woman who, with her husband out of town, invited me at 8:15 am into her hillside cottage—one of 25 in Santa Barbara designed by two notable women architects many years before. It was the best invitation I had had in years resulting in nothing more than a tour of the house! Still, there could have been more to walking that morning than walking . . .

". . . urban wanderings, delicious as they are, are not quite what we mean by walking. On pavements one goes by fit and start, halting to see, to hear, and to speculate. In the country one captures the true ecstasy of the long, unbroken swing, the harmonious glow of mind and body, eyes fed, soul feasted, brain and muscle exercised alike."

Christopher Morley, "The Art of Walking"

CHAPTER 12

SAND IN MY SHOES . . .

. . . "But the walking of which I speak has nothing in it akin to taking exercise..
but is itself the enterprise and adventure of the day."
—Henry David Thoreau

Some beaches have soft, deep sand making walking difficult even at the water's edge where beaches usually are more firm. Others are hard and easy to walk on. Some are volcanic black, some white, some pink.

Atlantic City's beach is unattractive. A dirty gray, it has a very long, gentle slope from the water's edge several hundred feet to the boardwalk. In spite of early morning daily tractor clean-ups it is more often littered than not. Still, the sand is hard near the water making it the easiest beach to walk on I've ever encountered. Black mussels attached to the huge black wooden supportive pilings add to the dark mystery of passing under the famous Steel Pier. It's a quiet time to fantasize how the not yet opened stores, restaurants, hot dog stands and amusement park rides above will soon bustle with activity. In the early morning a few elderly walkers, joggers and cyclists are on the boardwalk, but the famous wicker rolling chairs have yet to appear. A police patrol car drives slowly down the boardwalk while maintenance men repair broken boards and splinters caused by weather and the constant boardwalk traffic. In between famous old hotels and new gambling casinos are dozens of stand-up eateries, soft ice cream stores and cheap souvenir shops. It's not difficult even early in the morning to find an open store to grab a few pieces of Atlantic City's famous chewy salt water taffy.

In February 1943 I was sent to Atlantic City for Army Air Corps basic training. Nearly all the hotels were taken over for the GI's. The first three nights in the Air Corps I slept in the now demolished Chalfont Hotel main ballroom with 300 other soldiers. With only one bathroom to share, our bathroom shifts started at 3 am. Our daily routine included 6 to 8 hours a day of "hup-two-three-four" up and down the boardwalk in cold clear weather and in snow, sleet, and storm. One night, three weeks into my air corps incarceration, something happened which made me feel like a civilian again. After 8 hours of frigid marching there, at supper time, in the Chalfont mess hall, was the Glenn Miller Band! We listened in reflective joy and, after two weeks of eating nothing but peanut butter and bread to avoid adjusting to army food, the military cuisine that night tasted like steak.

Thanks to many overnight visits during New Jersey Broadcaster's Annual conventions I've had many down memory-lane morning walks in Atlantic City. Quietly I have tried a few "hup-two-three-fours" on my morning boardwalk saunters and belted out a few choruses of "Wait Till the Sun Shines Nellie," one of a dozen songs air cadets sang as they marched along. More than once passers-by have given me curious looks little realizing I was merely trying to recapture my 1943 marching rhythm.

One morning in 1984 I walked down to Convention Hall where, in February 1943, my first GI uniform and a pair of shoes two sizes too small were thrust upon me. It was 7:30 am as all the 1984 Miss America contestants were posing for photographers in bathing suits in front of Convention Hall. Hoping to go inside to recall the day I got my Government Issue, I was stopped at the door by a policeman. Still, watching America's most beautiful feminine scenery was superbly enjoyed for ten minutes.

We moved in and out of four hotels in four weeks in 1943. The first week from atop the seventh floor of the Lafayette Hotel our orders to "fall out!" precipitated a mad race seven floors downstairs to line up for the fearsome corporal in charge. Ex-boxer Corporal Joe from Jersey City then announced a GI party. It sounded like a thoughtful break in the routine.

As I walked by the Lafayette, I recalled that night when Corporal Joe issued buckets, brushes and strong chlorine smelling cleansers and told us to scrub all seven flights of stairs! At midnight our "GI party" was over when all but one of us had reached the seventh floor wiser and better adjusted to frustrating army routines. The exception was one complaining GI who was rewarded by being ordered to scrub his way upstairs with a toothbrush.

The front door of the New Belmont still opened on to the boardwalk. Now in 1984 it was a sadly neglected home for the elderly. It had already been an old dilapidated wooden hotel in 1943. Seven of us had been put in two small rooms connected by a bath. When we first entered our "suite" we casually noticed a "Quarantine—Measles" sign on the door. A week later when my parents paid me a Sunday visit, my mother noticed spots on my face. After they left, I hauled myself and all my belongings in a duffel bag off to the Haddon Hall Hotel which had been converted into an army hospital. Years later it became Atlantic City's first gambling casino, renamed Resorts International.

A quick diagnosis confirmed I had the measles. I then experienced one of those one-in-a-million encounters. My assigned hospital roommate, also with measles, was one of my best friends and next door neighbor in Bronxville, New York when I was 9 years old. We had not seen each other for 10 years and had a ball for the week we were quarantined.

Along with thousands of other GI's who had come for basic training, we had been marched to Haddon Hall on our second day of active duty. Forming two lines along a long hallway entrance that extended out to the broadwalk, we were pushed along into the hotel to be greeted by doctors and nurses on either side of us. "Roll up your sleeves, mister. BOTH arms." Then bing, bang, bong—on both arms—3 shots with needles the size of pencils! For days thereafter our arms were sore and many of us felt ill. Now, I walked along the Resorts long entrance hallway with shops on either side and illuminated signs pointing towards the casino. My vivid memories helped me reconstruct the scene as it had once been. I popped in a chocolate salt water taffy, left my hospital memories and continued my morning walk on the boardwalk along the beach.

Dudley and Polly and the Hoblers were touring in separate cars. We had enjoyed an overnight stay at a large former manorial home called Whitwell Hall Hotel a few miles from Castle Howard where the BBC "Brideshead Revisited" was filmed. As we separated after an English breakfast Polly waved goodby counseling us with an unfamiliar batch of names "maybe we'll see you tonight at the Tarn Inn in Talkin near Brampton in Cumberland." At dusk we encountered a vicious summer rain storm as we poked along a small one lane back road in our search for Talkin. The wind was fierce and the rain so hard it made visibility so limited we at first drove by the inn though it was only a few yards to our right. Dudley and Polly found the inn an hour later and joined us for an exceptionally fine candlelight dinner. Only three other people graced the quaint tiny dining room, one of whom was a Japanese gentleman. He somehow seemed out of character in this remote English Inn. At bedtime the storm continued unabated and I wondered how it might impede my morning walk.

By 6 am the storm had disappeared. Trees were down, debris was strewn about. There—right in front of this little inn—was a small lake— the tarn—which the storm had made invisible the night before. The water was absolutely calm. The pretty white beach around the lake had been beaten clean by wind and water. I took the footpath to the beach by crossing a pasture with munching sheep and cows.

The sky was now a striking clear blue. It was serenely quiet after the storm. At the far end of the lake a small bath house was nestled among a grove of pine trees. Several small 12 foot sailboats had been pulled up on the beach. Two dogs sat by the water's edge observing their stark naked master stride out of the water.

After completing a full circle of the lake back to the Inn, Polly and Dudley appeared ready to start their morning walk. My two-mile walk had been so peaceful and rewarding I volunteered to guide them around the lake. Excepting that the dogs and the naked man were gone, my second walk around was equally memorable this time enhanced by conversation with two good friends.

Our cottage was several hundred yards up the hill from the Coral Beach Tennis Club overlooking a magnificent coral pink Bermuda beach. Our four day 40th wedding anniversary trip was a surprise created by our three daughters. Daughter Debbie, a marathon runner, walked with me the first morning on the beach. The deep sand had a soft talcum powder texture making a gaited walk difficult and putting a strain on our calves. There was no surf and therefore no noise. We were alone until we saw a dog romping along side its master. They joined us to watch a sea level sunrise.

Daughter Mary Bassett walked with me the next day. We headed up hill on a road created by a huge cut through coral rock. As the early morning sun warmed up the pink and white Bermudian houses, the quiet and slightly cool temperature was similar to that wedding day forty years before on March 25, 1944 in San Antonio when I was an Air Cadet. It logically led to sharing some memories with Mary Bassett.

My bride-to-be with her father, mother and maid of honor had come from California by train. My father, mother, and sister had come from

New York. A special surprise was the unexpected arrival of my brother Wells who had commandeered an Air Corps plane to fly cross country to San Antonio from Stewart Field in Newburgh, New York where he was an instructor of West Point air cadets. He arrived with his new Captain's bars he'd received the day before.

The two dollar wedding license I had obtained at the county court house near the Hondo Air Base must have been designed in the 1850's. Larger than legal size paper, it had curlicues and old fashioned designs all over it. That Saturday morning I took off on the Hondo bus for an hour and half 50 mile bumpy trip past Texas sage brush and mesquite trees to San Antonio. We all met at the St. Anthony Hotel. To permit everyone to know each other a little better (albeit Randy and I had gone to school together from kindergarten through 7th grade and our parents knew each other), I sat with my in-laws-to-be at lunch, and Randy sat at a separate table with my parents.

Just before the wedding my father, apparently feeling a sense of responsibility as Best Man, and looking a bit embarrassed, asked, "Now, son, is there anything you'd like to know?" I suspected Dad correctly figured that I was still a virgin. However, not wishing to appear too innocent, I casually shrugged off his offer like a seasoned veteran and responded— "Thanks, Dad, I'm all set."

It was a small war-time wedding at St. Marks Episcopal church. An air cadet friend and his wife, two elderly locals, my in-laws and my mother were the only people in the church except for the wedding party: Maid of Honor Neill, my wife's best friend; Bridesmaid, my sister Ginny; Best Man, my father; Ushers, brother Wells, my best friend Wally who was engaged to Neill, and two temporary friends, fellow cadets who soon were to disappear from our lives. Right after the 12 minute service and a half dozen wedding photographs outside the church, my special wedding day gift to my bride arrived. Into a buggy we got as two horses took the newlyweds twice around the park winding up across from the church at the St. Anthony Hotel. All 14 of us then sat down in a private room for a wedding supper.

Now fully briefed on that great day 40 years before, Mary and I continued our Bermudian walk to the top of a hill and a magnificent view of the city of Hamilton across the sparkling blue-green waters of the bay. Ten minutes later, down near the water, a two horse buggy came clip-clopping along. I waved at the driver to stop to find out the cost of a one hour buggy ride.

And so, after a family lunch at the Four Ways Restaurant, I escorted Randy out the front door and there—very much like it had been 40 years before—was my surprise buggy and two horses. This time, we were not alone. We climbed into the buggy in the rear seats while daughters Debbie, Mary, and Nancy squeezed together in the front seat looking back at us. Off we all went for a happy one hour ride up and down the streets of Bermuda singing, laughing, taking pictures. The anniversary morning walk with my daughter had resulted in an unexpected anniversary present for my wife.

Ballachulish, about 75 miles northwest of Glasgow, is known as the locale of the Robert Louis Stevenson book "Kidnapped." Ardsheal House on Loch Linnhe was owned by a couple from lower New York State who spent 8 months a year in Scotland hosting guests from around the world. During the winter months he was chief steward of the Westminster Dog Show at Madison Square Garden.

Loch Linnhe is a narrow, 25-mile-long salt water bay that starts at the Firth of Lorne at the Atlantic Ocean and heads north north-east to Fort William. In between, sitting on a hill with a view perhaps four miles across the bay, is Ardsheal House. Most of this part of Scotland is rugged and sparsely populated.

Randy and I had joined eight other Princeton classmates for an October 1982 trip to Scotland. The first morning I looked out from my second story bedroom to check the weather. 400 yards away was Loch Linnhe covered with white caps under a gray, overcast day. Bundling up for the cool weather, I headed north past the garden and two palm trees that seemed out of place in this northern clime. After twenty minutes of exploring the hillside, it was downhill to the shore where, instead of an expected sandy beach, the shore was full of rocks and a preponderance of smooth egg-sized pebbles. The grass along the shore became my path since the beach was unwalkable. As the wind continued to increase in intensity the wind chill must have been at the freezing point. It was one of the few times in my thousands of walks that the weather caught me unprepared. I was COLD.

An obvious short cut to some barns took me through several fenced-in pastures. The country-boy in me concluded there would be a gate somewhere to the next pasture where cows were grazing. Now, there are at least three things to watch when crossing an occupied pasture. First, note whether the cows are horned or de-horned. Either way cows seldom cause problems for casual intruders. They usually keep their distance and stare at you curiously.

Second, bulls are not usually in the same pasture with cows but it can happen. For the city folk, the easiest way to tell the difference between horned cows and horned bulls is to notice what's hanging down between the rear legs. The one with four teats and the udder is the cow! In any event, size up the territory and quietly direct your feet away from any bulls in sight.

Third, watch where you step as you cross a pasture. Avoiding cow chips is a recommended caution. Look down to watch where you step—look up to watch for obtuse animals.

A few rain drops combined with the biting cold wind and the sight of two bulls caused me to pick up my pace to get quickly into the next pasture with its several dozen sheep. The sheep, unlike cows, were quite skittish and scampered off in all directions. This time I could see no gate at the end of the field and did not choose to climb the barbed wire fencing. Happily, one of those marvelous English "step-overs" came into view . . . a wooden stile with three steps up on one side, and three down on the other.

One pasture and one stile more brought me into the barnyard. The damp, dank, rich smell of cow manure encircled me. Immediately I was once again a farm boy shoveling manure on to a spreader on Dad's farm. For two summers as a teenager, I had milked cows, pitched manure, tossed hay and corn, cleaned out chicken houses, and weeded the vegetable garden. Putting in a 7 A.M. to 4 P.M. work day wasn't really my choice. Dad considered it good summer discipline for his youngest and sometimes rebellious son. By now it was raining and the already muddy barnyard was very slippery as I poked my head in a barn. In one stall were two small lambs and a ewe. Two very new calves were in an adjoining stall. A friendly extension of my hand to pet caused the calf to withdraw. Stroking the lamb was more successful. Now, a cat swooshed by chasing a mouse. A cackling chicken moved away from me. A shaggy old dog took off after the cat.

Forty-five minutes earlier I had set out with sneakers and a jacket prepared for a walk along the beach. Now, in the pouring rain, I was cold, my feet were wet and muddy. Still, all it took was a hot shower and a big breakfast to make the beginning of the day just perfect.

We were heading east from Dorset when I spotted a town on the map in Hampshire called Petersfield. The name triggered a vague recollection in my mind that Petersfield was where my great-grandfather Windsor had come from. Or was it great-great? And wasn't he a Congregational minister? The first church we located in Petersfield was the United Reformed Church. Yes, a lady advised, it once had been a Congregational Church and you'll find the pastor at his house some blocks away. Randy burrowed into a book in the car while the Rev. Cassingham served me tea after locating a very old, dog-eared ledger-size book of records. "I think the Windsors immigrated to the United States about 1845" I offered. He started his search in the 1830's when suddenly there they were . . . the names of three Windsors!

Back at the church we stood on the spot where the headstones had once been. The Windsors and all the other headstones had been in such disrepair that, with church and town approval, all had only recently been buried leaving only a plaque identifying the site as a former cemetery. (Upon my return home I not only confirmed that these Windsors were indeed my ancestors, but found a small cameo oil painting of two of them hanging on our living room wall.)

Thanks to that family research, we decided to spend the night in a Petersfield Bed and Breakfast within sight of a small lake. The next morning, after walking through part of downtown I headed out into some woods adjacent to a lake and a golf course.

The highlight of this walk, as has happened to me on numerous other occasions, was meeting not one, but TWO light colored Golden Retrievers. Unlike the darker color of most American Goldens, English Goldens are very blond, but share the same bounce, love, and smile from both ends as all Goldens all over the world.

Continuing around the lake I stopped to ask two fisherman about their luck. They had already caught several sunfish and two carp. A few hundred feet further, I stopped again to watch two ducks paddling along with seven ducklings trailing behind. The early morning sun sparkled on the water behind them.

The thrashing and churning of the water in some reeds at the water's edge caught my attention. It turned out to be a large school of carp. At breakfast with our hosts was another overnight guest, a young man from Germany who was hiking through England. His English was limited but as I related my morning walk, he smiled, seeming eager to hear more. His enthusiastically orchestrated responses either meant he was truly enjoying my little travelogue or he wasn't understanding a word. Either way, he made my day by listening.

One of the most impressive beaches I've ever seen is at Perrenporth, England in the western part of Cornwall. We had a room at a seaside boarding house overlooking the ocean. Hearing that the tides raced in and out, I checked tidal times and got up extra early the next morning. The beach was 2 to 3 miles long and shaped like a quarter moon. Excepting for Atlantic City, it was the widest and flattest beach I had ever seen. Standing at water's edge as the incoming tide moved rapidly, I stayed out of reach by moving a few steps at a time. Then, near where a river empties into the ocean, the water literally began racing in at an incredible pace. Within a short period of time what had been an expansive beach was only a small sliver of sand. It was an excellent walking beach that provided me the special fun of being a youngster at heart, alone on an expansive beach, and running away from the fast moving tide.

Palm Beach is a six mile long peninsula with the ocean on one side and Lake Worth, a salt water bay, on the other. The town is perhaps a quarter mile wide and as a result provides convenient beach walks and sunrises on the ocean side, or bike and walking path walks on the lake side.

The lakeside macadam path passes dozens of elegant homes, many with pools and high bushes to maintain privacy. The lawns and varieties of lush tropical growth are carefully manicured. Constantly patrolled by police cars, many of America's Gold Coast residents spend much of their time sharing their fortunes at charitable events or using their means to buy Cadillacs, Bentleys, Rolls Royces, or boats. They eat at their clubs and purchase clothes on Worth Avenue, the two block long extravaganza of expensive stores.

On the other hand ocean-side beach walks provide the walker an opportunity to see huge Palm Beach homes that cannot be seen from North County Road. While there is no direct access to the beach where the mansions are clustered, here and there are a few public access paths. During my one to three mile walks there were numerous opportunities to look at huge and ostentatious mansions some of which have been sold for $20 million or more.

After world-wide media reported a 200 foot long rusty ship had been blown ashore with its prow nudging the sea wall of the Joseph P. Kennedy home, I went out to inspect it. Two children with dad and mom were already walking under the rudder inspecting the decrepit ship. We exchanged speculation on the news report that the ship had been carrying drugs from South America.

Not even elitist Palm Beach can prevent man-made debris and dead Man-Of-War from washing ashore. In the water, these cloudy blue balloon-like creatures with long dangling tentacles sting upon contact. It hurts like the stab of a needle and can make you feel sick. I know, for I've been stung several times. Generally there are signs on the Florida beaches when Man-Of-War present a threat to swimmers. Most of the ones washed up on the beach are still balloon-shaped which will pop if you step on them. (Shoes are a requisite for this diversion.)

The Atlantic Ocean often provides excellent surf-boarding waves attracting early morning wet-suiters who coast in atop the waves on to the beach. Here and there the beach narrows making it almost impossible for the beach walker not to get wet feet as waves hit the shore. That presents a challenge to try to beat the surf and, as the waves recede, to dash across to the next dry spot before the waves return. Misjudging incoming waves can mean wet shoes and sandy socks, a small inconvenience for making beach walking more adventuresome. Still, a morning walk on any beach revives childhood memories of sand castles and swimming and family.

In early 1988, we went to Epcot and Disneyworld in Orlando for three days. It was there on February 24 that Gordon Fuqua from Jacksonville joined me for my 2000th consecutive before-breakfast morning walk. It was he who had started me on morning walking 6 years before while he was visiting our home in Princeton. To celebrate my milestone, we walked through the Polynesian Village Hotel grounds, across the street to the golf course where the Disney PGA golf tournament is held, around the Disney-made pond with real geese and ducks, and back along the small white beach at the edge of the Disney-made lake. The shell-less sand was hard and easy to walk on. We wound up on the dock where the Disney staff take fisherman of all ages out on the lake to seek Disney-stocked fish. To record my milestone, Gordon and I had our picture taken with the huge new Disney-duplicated Del Coronado Hotel in the background. No sea gulls, no shells, no pounding surf, but significant recognition of my 2000th consecutive day of walking before breakfast.

"There are three rules you have to follow. The first is, do whatever you want to do. The second is, do what you want to do, and the third is, do what you want to do." And so I was greeted by college roommate Ferd.

When Ferd was about 55, he came home one night to Princeton from New York, and decided he'd had enough of the "rat race." Thereupon he and Marge packed everything up and left a high pressure commuter lifestyle behind to live an enviable "on-the-beach" existence. Just south of Sarasota, Casey Key is a six mile long, very narrow island connected to the main land by a short bridge at either end. Part of their house had been a small decrepit military shed that they moved to the empty lot around which they had created a rustic style extension. The house is surrounded by tropical foliage with no view of water and is likely the only house on the key that does not face either the Gulf or the lake. It's like being a 1000 miles from civilization. They have a permanent open air bar on the ground floor as well as on the balcony by their bedroom. They and their guests always dress informally.

He completed his standard instruction for his guests, "Get up when you want. Skip a meal if you want. Say no to your host or hostess if you want. DO WHAT YOU WANT TO DO."

My umbrella kept me mostly dry the next morning from intermittent showers. The narrow gulf beach was more coarse than in other parts of Florida. Recent storms had left the water cloudy and brown. The winding, narrow two-lane road with its 15 mph speed limit took me past many different and mostly unpretentious homes. Judging by the license plates in the driveways, most residents were from northern climes. One man was tidying up his garage so I stopped to visit. Different size screws, nails, fuses. tools and whatnots were neatly organized above a workbench. I presumed him to be a man of precise talents and, sure enough, he was a science teacher from Chicago visiting his winter home for a month. He suggested I walk further north on Casey Key to see the *BIG* beach.

Along the *BIG* beach was the only development of new homes on the Key. The six or seven large houses were more like Palm Beach Gold Coast houses than the others on Casey Key. Many of the 600 homeowners on Casey Key were concerned about the opulence of these new homes in contrast to their generally more modest abodes.

At the *BIG* beach, there were no houses to disrupt an otherwise pristine beach scene. Traces of picnics and a small fire residue confirmed that others had recently enjoyed the scenery. A storm had created both a new inlet through the beach to the inner bay and a huge new dune fifty yards from the water. After ten minutes of sitting on the dune absorbing the tranquillity of the scene, I retraced the two miles back to my host's home. Since then I've done "whatever you want to do" two other times at the Baruches and always look forward to following that shoreline past attractive homes out to the *BIG* beach. It's like finding an old friend.

My first trip to Chicago was when my mother took me aboard a 21 passenger DC-2 at age 11 to the Chicago World's Fair in 1933. The Fair was located beside the lake not far from the present Hilton Hotel. Some of the buildings still remain. From most downtown Chicago hotels its not far out to the lake front and so during my walking streak I had walked several times along Lake Michigan both in winter and summer. January and February along the waterfront is a chilling wintry and windy experience.

One very cold February day I took a 25 minute walk toward the Fair site. En route I recalled a 1933 Worlds Fair attraction, a "modern" assembly line of tubes being filled with Ipana toothpaste. Then there was the wonder of the world's first streamliner train—the Burlington Zephyr! While this was an exciting 1933 sight, it paled by comparison to the outing a year later with my grandfather to see the same Zephyr roar through the countryside. People stood at road crossings waving at the engineers as the new miracle of streamlined railroad speed and comfort whizzed by. It was much like the early days of airplanes when the sound of a plane caused everyone to look skyward to see the miracle of flight. Now in 1987 along with several old engines and cars, the silver Zephyr was back on display in the middle of Soldiers Field where it once had first excited thousands of fair-goers in 1933.

Another recollection that morning was recalling the fair's luge-like ride down a winding water-rushing ramp. My mother sat behind me in the toboggan-like vehicle with me between her legs. We both screamed with excitement all the way down the twisting and turning ride that lasted three minutes. We promptly got right back up and did it over again.

A small plane convenience air strip is now a few hundred yards away from Soldiers Field by the same beach that I had walked with my family on a hot summer day in 1933. While the Ipana machine and toboggan ride were long gone, the observatory still remains. How exciting it was at age 11 to be creatively introduced to the stars and planets in a magic replica of the heavens. As I walked around the observatory in a biting wind 50 years later I vividly recalled that first introduction to the stars in 1933. Never could I have dreamed that twelve years later I would navigate by the stars in B-29 missions over Japan.

Neill, our maid of honor when we were married during my military service in 1944 in San Antonio, Texas, and her husband were living in Bodega Bay about 75 miles northwest of San Francisco overlooking the Pacific. A small village of 400 people, most have houses in and around the golf course on a mountainous foothill overlooking the ocean. Most every evening they sat in their living room watching multi-colored sunsets through a large picture window.

Each morning I'd walk a half mile down to the beach. It was firm and easy to walk on en route to the jetty two miles away at the entrance of Bodega Bay harbor.

Head down, a man seeking buried money or other metal walked slowly along guiding his metal detector in a search for hidden treasures. He stopped, dug into the sand, and came up with some loose change dropped by a careless bather. While the water was cold in April, a few yards away shoeless youngsters were gingerly testing the water. Suddenly with total abandon they ran all the way in with their clothes still on. Yells, screams and laughter confirmed the water was 54 degrees.

A man carrying a tote bag was carefully examining the beach. I asked him what he was looking for. "Sand dollars" he responded. "I hope I'm lucky enough to find one intact." Sand dollars look like a white seashell about the size of a 50 cent piece or silver dollar. Actually they are related to sea urchins. They break easily but in perfect condition are coveted as a beach treasure. He showed me four superb samples and moved on while continuing to stare intently down at the water's edge.

Small sandpiper birds with long bills walked rapidly along the beach ready to grab a fly or some small sea creature. Their thin spindly legs moved fast leaving delicate three-toed indentations on the sand. Fresh paw imprints suggested a dog had recently been frolicking with its master. Though some prints had been washed away by waves, some remained leaving tell tale signs of how the enthusiastic dog had suddenly changed direction and raced into the water.

I saw the opportunity to overtake another man with his Golden Retriever. "Huck" was a handsome male dog who was playfully rushing around. His owner turned out to be a writer and a former publisher who had moved from the east coast 11 years before. I told him about my proposed walking book. He gave me great encouragement and his business card with an offer to help once the book was done.

Forty minutes after my casual walk began, I arrived at the stone jetty where two youngsters were climbing over the rocks. Nearby two men, likely their fathers, were fishing. Something tugged at one line, the pole bent over and experienced hands smoothly started cranking in the line at the end of which was a crab. "Good eating" he said as a fishing boat passed through the channel. Looking back east towards the hills—over two miles away—I could see low hanging clouds over my host's house. The sunrise there was always unusual as the hills to the east blocked the sun for a half hour after Bodega Bay and the ocean was in daylight. Suddenly, the sun popped over the hills. It was time to retrace my steps.

There were two sets of shoe prints in the sand. One set seemed to have been left by a woman or a small man. The other was obviously a jogger for the distance between strides was longer. I decided to walk in the footsteps of the one set that seemed more equal to my stride. Whoever he was, he had not walked in a straight line for while placing my feet in his steps I staggered left and right until the shoe prints disappeared at water's edge. Seeing no exit footprints from the water I fantasized what could have happened to him.

The wide beach challenged me to close my eyes. Could I walk as confidently and in a straight line? I closed my eyes and walked with confidence for 10 paces. After 20 paces I had to open my eyes. Then I went 30 paces, then 40. Suddenly my feet got wet. Opening my eyes I saw I had veered too far and was at the oceans edge. Once again I realized how much confidence a blind person must acquire to walk with balance and a sense of direction.

Poipu Shores is on the western part of one of the most beautiful tropical islands in the world. Our friends the Worthingtons visit the Hawaiian Island of Kuaui each winter for several months and frequently host friends. From a small porch off their third floor condo living room they have a front row seat to enjoy the sight and sound of crashing waves against the lava rocks below. Watching the sun each evening as it disappears into the western ocean adds an emotional ingredient to the happy hour no bartender can mix.

One morning I headed north through Poipu village past a small beach protected by a narrow sandbar that extended out several hundred yards. Happily the tide was out so I could walk almost all the way out on the sandbar and get a view back to the shore. I next found a back entrance to the Sheraton Hotel and wandered through the lobby, past shops, the dining room, and the pool. Just beyond the hotel was a large cactus garden with a dozen narrow garden walkways which wound through an incredible variety of small and large cacti. Further along the shore, was a bluff that provided me a look down into a huge cavern 60 feet below. Waves were crashing inside with an echoing roar throughout the cavern.

A few minutes later I watched some early bird golfers teeing off and then found myself on the edge of a huge volcanic hole perhaps 500 yards across. Below in the caldera were 30 houses and several tennis courts. While protected from the wind, the residents had no view. Still, it had to be better than winter weather back home.

After leaving Kuaui, we spent the night at the famous Royal Hawaiian Hotel in Honolulu. Our room on the third floor overlooked Waikiki Beach with Diamond Head off to our left. The afternoon before we had seen thousands of people on the beach, outrigger canoes riding the surf, small sailboats rented from beach hotels bouncing along between the waves, and surfers swimming out with and riding back on their surfboards.

This early morning the beach was being raked by tractor and touched up by hand. Life guards and hotel employees were putting out lounge chairs by the pool side, straightening up centerboard sailboats, filling in beach holes and without apparent remorse leveling away a sand castle some youngster had built the day before.

My walking route took me into in the Moana Hotel where we had stayed during our first visit to Hawaii with our daughter and son-in-law in 1974. It, and the adjoining Royal Hawaiian, are the two oldest hotels on the beach. I stopped to look at old photographs along the hallways capturing the 1920's atmosphere of both hotels when early cruise ships were the only mode of transportation to Hawaii.

Now it was 7:30 and dozens of walkers were on the beach. Seemingly most of these tourists were from Japan. Thinking of Pearl Harbor and my B-29 missions over Japan, it was strange to realize the economy of the 50th state now relied heavily on the invasion of Japanese tourists. I bowed slightly to a young Japanese couple and completed my walk.

The dozens of walks I've had along the peaceful and majestic shoreline at La Jolla, California would never have happened except for Major Tremper Longman. He looked about 50 when our Lieutenant snapped us to attention at the Santa Ana Army Air Base in 1943. Following the Major's welcome to Classification ("We will determine here whether you will be a pilot, bombardier or navigator"), we were dismissed.

With bravado unknown to most cadets fearful of officers I approached the Major, snapped to in a brace, saluted and said "Cadet Herbert W. Hobler, Sir. Sir, by any chance sir, do you have a son, sir, who went to Princeton, sir?" Indeed his son was Tremper Longman Jr. Our brief conversation ended with his offer "If I can be of any help, Cadet Hobler, please feel free to come see me." A parting salute, a quick about face, and off I went while several friends watched in amazement that their buddy Hobler had actually approached a Major.

Ten days later I was ordered to The Major's office. What had I done? Expecting an impersonal military chastisement or worse he astounded me with "Hobler, you're on orders to be shipped out to Texas. However, if you would prefer to stay here in Santa Ana, just let me know." I couldn't believe my ears but promptly responded "Sir, I have friends here, sir, and if I had my choice sir, I would stay here, sir."

Major Longman then got on a squawk box and told his aide "Take Hobler off orders to Texas and assign him to stay here at Santa Ana." That weekend I looked up a La Jolla girl I had gone to school with back east from kindergarten through the 7th grade. It took just 7 short weekend dates for Randy and me to get engaged.

As our four youngsters grew up whenever we could afford it, we took them west to La Jolla to see their grandparents. It didn't take long to develop the same affection and love my wife had for beautiful La Jolla by the sea. Long after her parents had died we continued to be refreshed with the charm of La Jolla by spending a night or two at the old La Valencia Hotel.

La Jolla is appropriately translated as "the jewel." Tall palm trees line the park walk along the ocean. A promontory called Alligator Head overlooks a small beach widely known as "the Cove." A hundred yards to the south is a rugged shoreline, almost always with crashing and exploding waves. Looking to the north, the California coastline can be seen for miles and miles. To the east are hundreds of lovely homes nestled in the hills above the village.

The frequent early morning fog over La Jolla soon burns off. Whether foggy, overcast or under the usual sparkling clear blue sky, the La Jolla shore always attracts early morning walkers. Brisk walkers outnumber the slower pace of many elderly people. For every age there's always the fascination at low tide of a descent down to the rocks to watch marine life scurrying in tidal pools–little minnow size blennies, sea anemones, snails, hermit crabs and long strands of kelp that have washed ashore. Adding to the sights is a healthy stimulating salt water seaside smell.

A walk along the La Jolla shore is the ultimate morning stroll—a good ocean smell, the sun coming up at your back, the alternate sound of quiet then crashing waves, the exploration of sea life, stepping on kelp pods for an explosive sound, the freshness of a balmy crisp morn. It's a "good-to-be-alive" experience. Little did Major Longman know what he did for me when he changed my military orders in 1943.

Fourteen Princeton classmates and their wives flew to Lisbon in 1984 the day after our 40th reunion unified with luggage stickers reading, "A '44 Thrill in Estoril." A charter bus took us to the small southwestern coast town of Estoril known for its gambling casinos and beautiful shores.

At 6:15 am the first morning I went across the railroad tracks to the rocky beach to encounter a pleasant sea smell. While the beach was quite walkable I got off it onto a concrete sidewalk between the beach and a parallel wide highway and headed west to find Cascais two miles away. A New York friend had told me it was a charming town that had a particularly outstanding restaurant.

At the edge of town situated fifteen feet above the edge of the water was The Albatroz. At 7:00 a.m. it was not yet open for reservations so I enjoyed ten minutes of window shopping through the picturesque village before heading back towards the water. A small boat was being pulled up on the beach, and a dog leaped out as a fisherman hauled out several boxes and headed towards what turned out to be the fish market building. I realized what was about to happen, for several years before while visiting my nephew David in Honolulu he had talked me into going to a 5:30 a.m. fish auction. Now here inside this Portuguese building were hundreds of mackerel, sea bass, tuna and shrimp being displayed. A piece of paper on each fish identified its owner. Standing around waiting to see what price their fish would bring were fifteen to twenty crusty old fisherman with a few younger, deeply tanned associates. Five or six fishermen-to-be youngsters moved in close to watch the auction as two dogs peered in through the open doorway. There was a strong but good smell of fish. The auctioneer began spewing out weights and prices in rapid Portuguese as a confederate pointed out the particular fish being auctioned.

The bidders were restaurant owners and retail store buyers. As a fish was bought, the auctioneer's assistant scribbled information on a sales list. How the owner got paid, how the buyer got his fish and paid for it was a mystery to me though obviously they all knew what they were doing. The characters in my morning drama were following routines that had been played out for generations. Seldom had I ever stopped during my morning walk for more than a few minutes but this auction spectacle kept me absorbed for twenty minutes.

Two interesting things occurred on the sidewalk back to Estoril. As a train raced by on my left and ocean waves crashed on the beach on my right, a young couple approached. I chose to start a conversation.

"I presume you are Americans. How long are you going to be here?" The man introduced himself as Phil Whitcomb. "Only for one day. We both work for TWA and came over on the airline just for the weekend at practically no cost. How could we refuse?" Responding to my identification that Princeton, N.J. was my home we found we had a mutual friend that led to several minutes of conversation.

This chance encounter once again strengthened my habit for frequently opening up conversations with strangers.

A half mile beyond I had almost reached the train station in Estoril when three young men blocked my passage. As I started to go around them, all three moved in front of me. One said, "Hey mister, got a light?" I said I didn't. Then one of them flicked off my cap. Not sure of their intentions and with no one else in sight, I pretended to be casual in picking up my cap and moved on. After crossing the railroad tracks I cautiously turned to make sure they were not pursuing me.

I have ventured in back alleys and strange places without concern many times on my walks. Perhaps my imagination got the better of me, but this time I had been truly concerned and was delighted to get back to my room. At breakfast with classmates I recounted my walk to Cascais and locating the Albatroz Restaurant, watching the fish market auction, meeting the TWA weekenders with common friends, and my three "punks" encounter. While they had slept, my hour and a half early walk had once more given me an adventurous head start on the day.

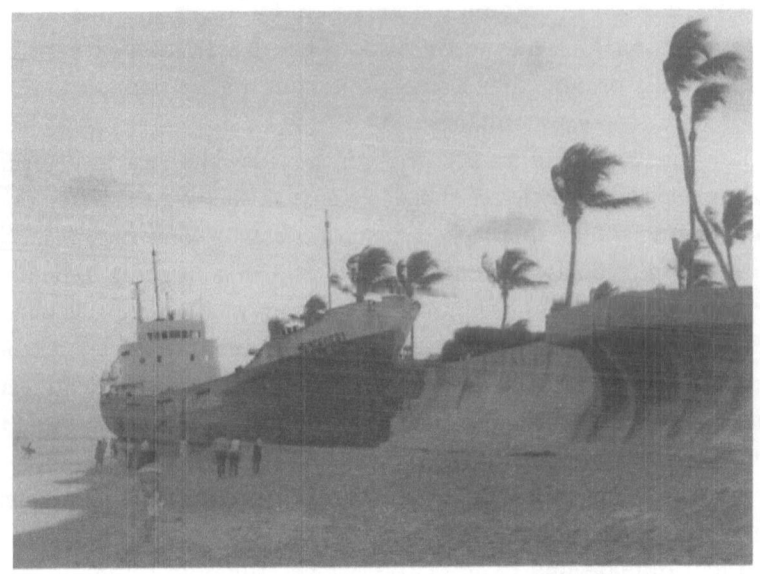

Nicaraguan ship, J. F. Kennedy beach, Palm Beach
Dec. 1984

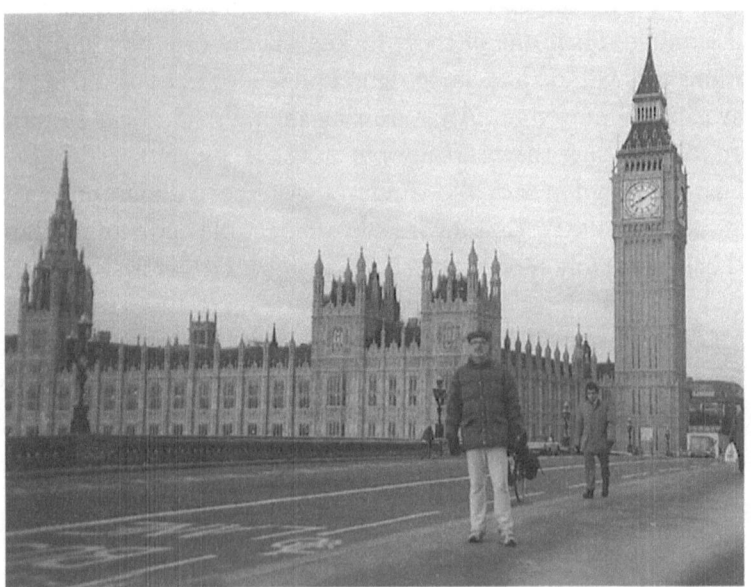

8:10 a.m., Big Ben, London
January 22, 1986

POSTSCRIPT

I realize few of my readers might ever enjoy such an exotic trip as my wife and I took in 1991. It was a once-in-a-lifetime experience for us which provided me many rare morning walks that I'd like to share with you.

THE ULTIMATE:
A WALK AROUND THE WORLD

The expensive brochure promised a trip around the world in a private jet. The color photos of exotic places were tantalizing, the luxury seemed unbelievable, and the mere idea of a first class trip around the world in a huge private jet was almost incomprehensible. We set the brochure aside when we saw the price.

A year later a similar brochure arrived. We were over sixty-five, and when some one reminded us of the adage "If you don't spend it your children will" we signed aboard.

Normally seating 300 people, the L1011A had been redesigned for 80 first class seats, a bar and two lounges. A young and attractive crew of 16 was aboard to wait hand and foot on us for the 35 day, 40,000 mile trip that started in Miami. On *DAY ONE* 8 hours after our first take off we landed in Santiago, Chile.

The next morning was a cool 48 degrees at 6:40 am. Few people were in sight. I passed by a beautifully manicured park along the river, stopped midway on a bridge to watch the roaring dark brown silted river beneath, and a few blocks beyond stopped in front of a supermarket. I went in to compare food and prices back home. It had a feeling of a vintage 1950 U.S. supermarket with narrow aisles, few frozen foods, lots of canned foods, a less than attractive fresh vegetable display and no automatic equipment at the check-out counter. There were a few U.S products. Interestingly, after converting pesos to dollars, the prices seemed lower than those than back home.

The return walk to the San Cristobal Hotel took me through a residential neighborhood reminiscent of California homes except that virtually every home had front yard metal fences with locked gates. Further evidence of an obvious safety concern were the bars over the first floor windows. Lilacs and yellow bushes were everywhere evident inside the small front yards. On a pole 3 feet high at the curbside of each home was an open basket-like metal container into which garbage bags were placed. The novel idea made it easy for pick up while being safely out of reach of roaming dogs.

For me the highlight of the trip started on day DAY FOUR on Easter Island. 2500 miles west of Santiago, this 7 by 15 mile Chilean island is home to 2800 people mostly of Polynesian descent. Isolated from the world, there are now two commercial flights a week landing on the longest airstrip in the world. (It was built by NASA in 1967 as an emergency landing strip for space shuttles.) Tourists first arrived in 1967 and the natives, catering to the new island visitors, imported the Hawaiian hula to entertain them. Originally discovered on Easter Sunday in 1772 by Capt. Edward Davis, the natives call their island the navel of the world as no other civilization exists within any 2500 mile direction.

As my walk started and the sun rose, the Chilean Diuca birds sang their morning welcome along the dirt road. The black lava shore was being pounded by waves as I encountered a sweet honeysuckle-like smell permeating the air. A rooster crowed as a small fishing boat turned off its engine and glided into a small inlet where fishermen began unloading their early morning tuna catch. No one paid attention to me as young boys and old men joined in tossing fish on the dock.

A few hundred yards further the sight of the tops of white crosses ahead telegraphed the location of a cemetery. Each grave was bounded by a rectangular border of black basalt or volcanic tuft, now painted white. Wild flowers were growing around most graves. A few wooden crosses contained names and dates of the deceased. Weathering had rapidly erased the vital statistics of many wooden crosses as well as those made of concrete which had crude hand painted names and dates. It was obvious no identification of the late beloved would be readable after three or four years. One touching section of the little cemetery were small plots and small crosses exclusively for children.

A quarter mile beyond was an ahu, a sacred site with a lava stone base on which stood five large Moai statues. Having seen a PBS-TV special about these 20 to 80 ton statues 8 to 15 feet high, it was thrilling to be on Easter Island to see and touch them. All five faced inland, originally placed there to honor a village chieftain. The huge basalt figures that once had huge white eyes now had empty black sockets.

Peter Edmunds, our native island guide, was an exceptionally talented and educated man who had received college and MBA degrees at UCLA. After ten years he had chosen to leave California smog and the complications of an industrial nation to return to the simplicity of Easter Island. He took us to a mountainous hill where the island's 827 widely dispersed statues had once been carved. The mystery had always been how natives could possibly have moved 50 or 70 ton statues down the mountain across the island to a permanent site. Peter suggested a logical answer as he showed us an almost completed chiseled-out statue still lying on its back in the side of the mountain. By placing round stones under the body to act like ball bearings, the natives pulled the statue out from the side of the mountain until it fell feet first into a deep pit. Now the huge standing statue was ready to be "walked" down the hill inch by inch with stone ball bearings beneath its feet and ropes to control its upright balance. It sounded like a logical albeit an incredibly creative solution.

Tahiti was our next stop where our airplane crew joined us for four days aboard the Windsong. A new four hundred foot, four masted engine driven cruise ship, its full complement of sails (raised and trimmed by computer) added both beauty and smoothness to its movement.

Next morning on DAY EIGHT, the rising sun peeking through dark clouds combined with a warm tropical breeze and the relaxed movement of the ship provided me an intoxicating wake-up experience. Behind the ship were the disappearing flickering night lights of Tahiti while 30 miles ahead on the dawning horizon was the island of Raietea. With not a soul stirring at 5:30 am, the nine-laps-to-a-mile ship was all mine to experience an exquisite south Pacific fantasy walk. Twenty-five exhilarating laps later now with an almost indiscernible Tahiti to the stern, Raietea ahead loomed ever larger. It was Sunday and ashore stores were closed as we bounced along on wooden seats in the back of a converted truck, the closest thing to a bus the islanders could provide. The most memorable thing about our four hour visit was to learn that the native language consisted of 5 vowels and 8 consonants.

The next morning lap after lap around the ship I could see Bora Bora came closer and closer with the spectacular Mt. Otenamu dominating the entire island. Little wonder it became known as the fabled Bali Hai. Mt. Otenamu grew in size until we passed right by it before dropping anchor.

Our one day visit included a 22 mile open air bus trip—again in a truck-converted bus—from Vaitape around the Bora Bora shores on unpaved roads. Most houses were tidy and small with corrugated metal roofs. Our guide pointed out mangos, breadfruit, banana, taro, sweet grapefruit, papayas, coffee, a lazy hibiscus, Kapok and coconut trees. The fabled copra, once an important coconut by-product, now was no longer exported. Hardly a trace of the huge American World War II naval base was left though the lagoon that harbored dozens of WWII Navy ships was easily identified.

Having experienced two delectable sun rise approaches to Raietea and Bora Bora, could there be one more the third morning? Directly ahead of the ship clouds hung over the tops of a mountainous profile as the sun rose on *Day Nine* directly behind Moorea. After every three minute lap, the scenic view from the bow towards Moorea was constantly changing as small clouds disappeared, large clouds changed shapes and the rising sun bounced off different hills. Anticipating a new scene after each lap I picked up my pace so as to round the stern more quickly to return to the bow. These 35 laps created 35 never-to-be-forgotten changing post card scenes of the most beautiful of the three islands discovered by Capt. Cook in 1769. An island of ironwood and Caribbean pine trees, dense foliage, pineapple plantations and towering jagged mountains, it also was the site for filming "Mutiny on the Bounty" with Marlon Brando in Cook's Bay. Brando's twin over-the-water thatched roof cottages were worth a photo.

Port Douglas in Australia is one hour north of Cairns, an hour away by boat from the Great Barrier Reef. The new Mirage Hotel consisted of six separate three story white buildings all with a view of the ocean and each surrounded by swimmable lagoons. The clean three to four mile long beach provided me three exceptional morning walks as the sun rose directly to the east over the water. On *Day Eleven* I walked north two miles into the village of Port Douglas itself. The newly built harbor in a town described as Australia's emerging Palm Beach, provided me close up inspection not only of yachts, but of several large high speed hydrofoil boats that carry up to 200 people out to the Great Barrier Reef an hour out into the ocean for a snorkeling experience second to none in the world. The doors to a new indoor shopping mall adjacent to the piers were open permitting me an interior walk to window shop before heading back.

A cemetery by the roadside with no fencing and some old headstones prompted me to stop for an inspection. How could they be old in such a young country? The headstone engravings provided some of the answers. "Died at sea, August 15, 1886," "A seafarer for 30 years, died age 55 July 6, 1894," "Shot and killed in Billy's Bar October 15, 1888" told its own story of life in a seafaring village. Most of the concrete, wood, and metal headstones were well preserved. Stone apparently was not native to this sandy area.

It's not often I've walked without shoes but the last day off came my shoes and into the edge of the ocean water went my feet. The mildly breaking waves and warm water created a luxurious, splashing, two mile walk.

We had visited Hong Kong six years before. This time our hotel was in Kowloon across the bay from Hong Kong. Our 8th floor view from the Shangri La provided a spectacular daytime view of ships moving in all directions between Kowloon and the fantastic skyline of multi-colored skyscrapers on Hong Kong. At night the movement of lights aboard ships combined with the millions of lights stretching from the top of Hong Kong's mountain down to the water level made it even more breathtaking.

On DAY FIFTEEN I walked from the Shangri La along the waterfront past the Regent, the Peninsula and other well known hotels, crossed some busy streets and arrived at the Star Ferry. One Hong Kong dollar bought me a lower level ticket. (Two dollars provides access to the upper level.) As the gate for the next ferry opened, hundreds of mostly Chinese rapidly moved aboard and sat down on benches amidship. Some read newspapers while others sat and stared in what obviously for them had become a boring daily commuting routine.

The seven minute ferry ride provides a dramatic view of both Hong Kong ahead and Kowloon behind, as well as a front seat to watch what best can be described as a dodge 'em game. Needing to compensate for strong currents, hundreds of small boats, ferries, large ships, and junks constantly darted this way and that as if they were playing a game of maritime chicken.

At 6:30 am Hong Kong was already bustling with activity as I stopped in to visit the lobby of what some call the world's finest hotel–the Mandarin. An hour and a half after departing from the Shangri La I had enjoyed two ferry rides, picked up an International Herald Tribune, located a camera store for later shopping, rubbed elbows with thousands of Chinese, passed many Caucasians walking or jogging along the water front path, and finished the last 10 minutes with an elderly fellow Jet Tour passenger who was out to "get my morning constitutional." It was 8:15 on my 3266th consecutive day of walking before breakfast.

Now in India, we were to take a 6:15 am "bullet" train on Day Eighteen from New Delhi to Agra to see the Taj Mahal. The alarm was set for 3:45 am. I had no reason to believe a walk was unsafe and walked 10 to 15 blocks from the hotel past two story apartment buildings, private homes and a small park. It was warm, extremely quiet and uncrowded. The smog and musty air-polluted atmosphere was due not just to heat and trapped bus and car pollution, but because so many Indians cook with cow chips. An entrance to a golf club piqued my curiosity so I walked in the drive to inspect the first tee and the outside of the small clubhouse. No one was in sight.

After breakfast at 5:15, the train left at 6:15. Two hours later we were in front of the majestic Taj Mahal. Built by Shah Jahan from 1631 to 1653 with 20,000 workers, it was a tomb for his 39-year-old wife Mumtaz Mahal who died after her 11th child. He was to lay beside her after he died in 1658. A simulated tomb of the two is under the dome on the main floor. The more adventuresome tourist can inch down a steep set of stone stairs to the real tomb below. It is a hot, stifling chamber best promptly vacated after a quick view of the sepulcher.

The next day, a Saturday, I stopped by the golf course again, this time about 6:30 am. Like many popular American public courses, there was an early foursome on the first tee with several other foursomes waiting their turn. Unlike American golfers, some were dressed in native Indian style dress, some turbaned, some bearded. For a Westerner, at least, it was an extraordinary golfing sight.

Jetting around the world next took us on Day Twenty to Mahe in the Seychelles, a lovely group of islands 1000 miles east of Kenya. 60,000 people on 116 islands speak mostly their native Creole along with French and English.

The 85-90% year-round humidity was bearable that first morning thanks to an off-shore breeze. Two morning walks took me along a very white beach, through a jungle-like lush tropical foliage to explore where natives lived, then up a long hill to a little village to stop at St. Francis Catholic Church. This particular morning, five young girls dressed in white were gathering for their first communion. They carried colorful flowers, had lace veils, and were escorted by very dressed-up parents.

Mahe is full of purple, red and white Bouganvilla and sweet smelling gardenia trees. No more was this evident than behind the Plantation Club, our beachfront hotel for three days. A small pond there was bordered with coral palisades, palm trees, and floating lily pads. It was as if a Hollywood set designer had created it for Dorothy Lamour.

Capetown, South Africa rates highest on my list of the most beautiful cities in the world. Much like San Francisco, it is clean, its temperatures moderate (the same latitude as North Carolina or San Diego). The city is magnificently nestled between Table Mountain behind and the ocean in front. Its people are friendly and the wide streets are bordered with abundant trees, flowers and shrubs. First settled in 1652 by a Dutchman, French Huguenots followed in 1688 and the British in the 19th century. Diamonds were discovered in 1866 and gold in the 1870's starting what eventually would be one of the best economies in the world.

My daily pre-breakfast Capetown walks were uphill into mixed architectural residential sections reminiscent of California and New York, and then downhill into the main part of the city. Much of the city looks new though some buildings must be 75 to 100 years old. A path through the mile long narrow park from our Mt. Nelson Hotel to center city passes the South African Museum, Parliament, and statues of Cecil Rhodes and Jan Christian Smuts. The former, whose fortune came mainly from diamonds, would rank among today's richest men were he still alive. He plowed much of it back into the development of South Africa. The latter was a great South African General and statesman of the early part of the 20th century.

I walked into the city, went underground via a long escalator to find a city beneath the city. An area of perhaps 6 or 8 blocks square had recently been created below ground as a shopping mall with access routes to numerous parts of the city. My escalator exit brought me up into a very modern railroad station and the lobby of a high office building. Having taken the cable car ride to the top of Table Mountain behind the city the day before, this morning I then walked a mile uphill as far as streets would allow to be within a short distance of the cable car origination point. I paused to absorb two exceptional views, one to the city stretched out below and the other almost straight up to the Table Mountain Bluff.

The Blue Train is a 24-hour elegant facility between Capetown and Johannesburg. As I had done on a somewhat similar trip on the Orient Express, up to the engine and back I went, through the train to the last car, back and forth for two miles. There was time to look out wide windows at flat land and mountains, at high mounds of leftover dirt from gold and diamond mines, and, as we came into Johannesburg, at hundreds of shacks into which huddled thousands of "free" blacks searching for jobs and new opportunities.

After a six hour visit by bus throughout Johannesburg with its thousands of lavender jacaranda trees, we were jetted to Nairobi for a night at the Safari Park Hotel. My walk the next morning was an unexciting three trips around the grounds. The next morning we had a one hour flight in a CD-3 to start a safari.

During the briefing of what and what not to do in the Masai Mara Safari Village, it became evident this was one place I would not venture far on my walk. We were told a stray elephant, hippopotamus, lion and baboon had more than once wandered through our encampment. Indeed, Kaka, the natives' name for a particular stray elephant, walked into our breakfast area one morning and, after we had judiciously removed ourselves to a more protective area, he trunked a plate and napkin off the table before grabbing a few rolls. That night a native with a protective speer came into our dining tent to lead us back to our sleeping tent and there munching grass 30 feet away was a hippopotamus. The next day while we were out in Land Rovers watching animals, two baboons broke into a neighbor's tent to spirit away food that should not have been left in the tent.

Judiciously, I restricted my morning walks to the compound.

For two days we bounced in Land Rovers over the savanna watching lions devour gazelles and wildebeest (with hyenas ready to move in on the remains as vultures stood by). We were lucky to spot the normally elusive leopard that has dragged its kill up in a tree. We watched a cheetah stalk a stray zebra, listened to water explosions as dozens of hippos rose up out of the Mara River a few feet from a sleepy looking crocodile, and enjoyed the sight of small herds of adult and baby elephants and clusters of two or three gentle giraffes.

The third morning I wakened early at 5:15 to get in a mile and a half walk around the compound before our native Askari warrior rapped at our tent flap at 5:50 am. He still had his flashlight and protective club handy to escort us through the semi-darkness to breakfast. After a ten minute Landrover ride with Sam, our native guide, we groped our way down 20 steps to the edge of the Mara River. There 8 of us were packed into a flat bottom boat that tippily was pulled by rope across to the other side. A hundred yards beyond were three yet-to-be-filled hot air balloons. Soon 12 of us climbed up into a basket which held 3 people in each corner compartment. The jet flames began blasting hot air into the enlarging balloon. With the pilot in the middle we were ready for take-off.

It was DAY TWENTY-NINE at 6:30 in the morning as we rose into absolute quiet under a clear sky with the sun rising above the horizon to the east. Up to two hundred, then five hundred feet, then down to three hundred feet and lower as we gazed below at roving elephants, zebras, water buffalos, wildebeests, giraffes and lions. Behind us two other colorful balloons silently moved in contrary elevations to add to the scenic spectacle. An hour later we eased down to the ground, the basket turning on its side with a mild jar.

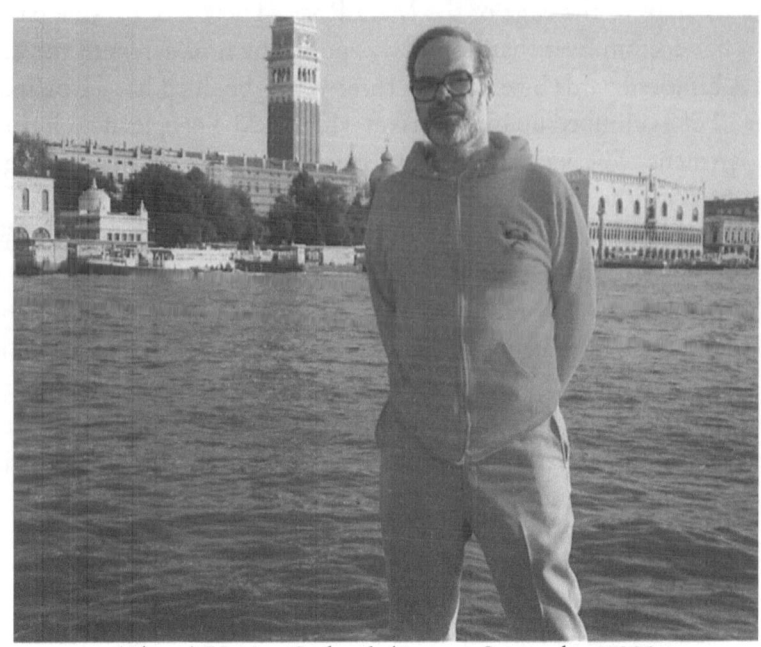

(Above) Venice, Italy, 6:45 a.m., September 1983.
(Below) Taka visits at breakfast, Masai Mara Reservation, Kenya
November 1991

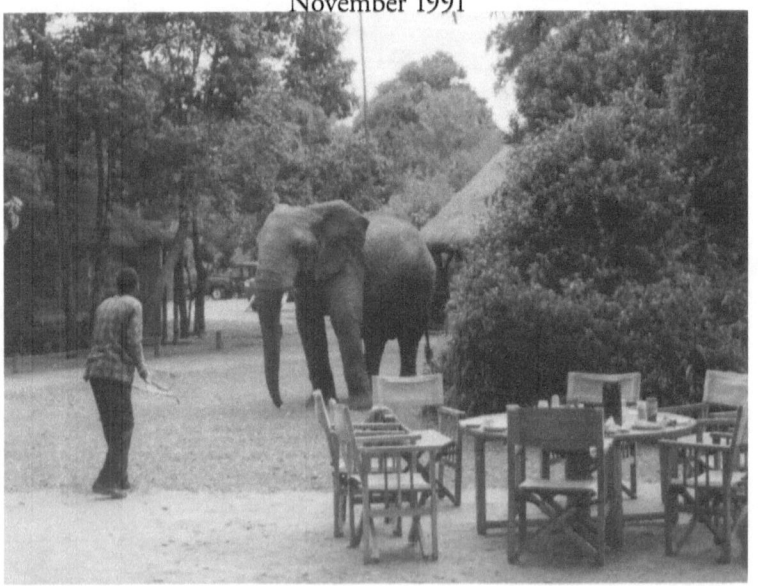

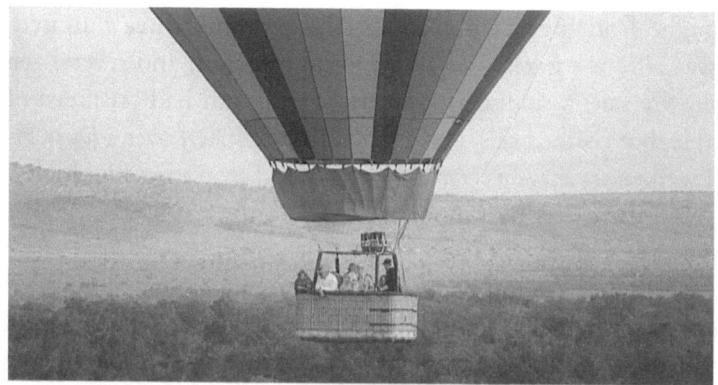

6 a.m. Sunrise above the animals, Kenya, November 1991

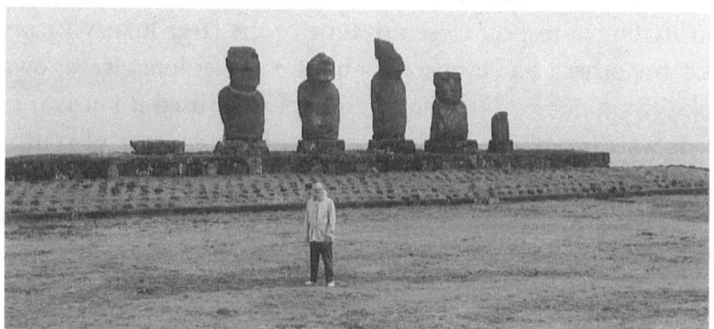

Easter Island statues, October 1991

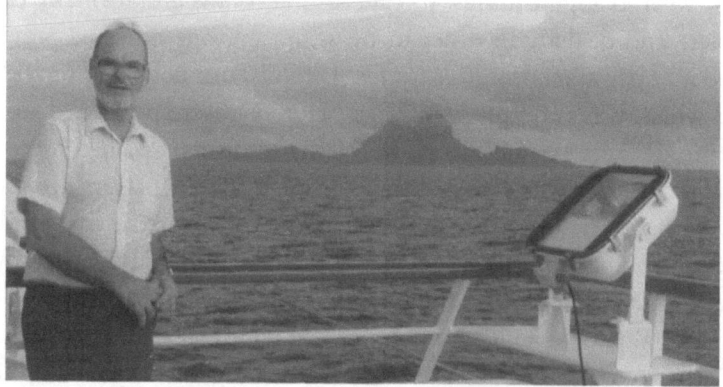

Shipboard sunrise at Bora Bora, October 14, 1991

A hundred yards away was an advance Landrover staff preparing our breakfast at a long portable eighteen inch high table. As we sipped champagne from pewter goblets on the savanna, three hundred yards away was a lion, a gazelle in the opposite direction and several zebras in another. We sat on six-inch high canvas seats and had breakfast of fresh pineapple, hot coffee, rolls, and French toast cooked over a jet burner hot plate. I walked seventy-five yards away to stand atop a five foot high termite hill. Could there ever be a more out-of-the-ordinary, elegant, exotic early morning experience?

Our jet tour around the world was about to end, but not before spending three nights at the Hotel de Paris in Monte Carlo. If Capetown is not the most beautiful city in the world then Monte Carlo is. Certainly it exudes wealth.

One morning I walked down the hill from the hotel into the semi-circular harbor to inspect close up some of the large luxury yachts. One dwarfed any other I had ever seen. About 340 feet long, it was owned by a Greek tycoon named Niarchos who I was told used it but two months a year. It was incomprehensible to think of the expense of staffing and maintaining it. Another morning I walked into town and up a hill to the palace of Prince Ranier where a round-the-clock sentry stands at informal attention. Even more reflective for me was to enter the nearby cathedral where Princess Grace is entombed.

The famous Casino was next to our hotel. That night, thinking I might play some blackjack at $2.00 a chip, Randy joined me to inspect the opulent facility with its high ceilings, private dining rooms and formally dressed croupiers and dealers. In order to be admitted, one must be previously cleared and pay a handsome entry fee. Happily, our hotel had provided us a pass which was carefully scrutinize before we were permitted to enter. Chermin de fer is a gambling game I didn't understand. There were three dealers with one sitting elevated above some fifteen players around the table. With a little imagination it was easy to presume the cast of players included—Sidney Greenstreet, Peter Lorre, Humphrey Bogart, Edwardo Cianelli, Charlie Chan, and the Dragon Lady. It was an amalgamation of international people none of whom looked happy or trustworthy. After a fascinating ten minutes of watching card dealing and chips being tossed here and there, we inspected the roulette room, the craps room, and finally found two blackjack tables. The minimum $100 chip destroyed my hope of claiming to have gambled in this famous Monte Carlo casino. Down the street I found another casino with $5 chips.

My once-in-a-lifetime 35 pre-breakfast walks around the world had only covered 160 miles. Still, lest one think my morning walks were thereafter forever spoiled, my best walk in 36 days was that first morning home on familiar territory with my loving Golden Echo.

www.ingramcontent.com/pod-product-compliance
Lightning Source LLC
Chambersburg PA
CBHW020901310526
45786CB00018B/572